Table of Contents

Red Grapefruit Smoothie

Raspberry Red Lettuce Smoothie

Cranberry Red Leaf Lettuce Smoothie

50 Shades of Smoothies

Frozen Berries Smoothie

Superfoods Smoothie Popsicles

Pomegranate Watermelon Smoothie

Orange Carrot Smoothie

Carrot Orange Papaya Smoothie

Carrot Pumpkin Smoothie

Raspberry Cauliflower Smoothie

Pomegranate Yogurt Smoothie

Mango Papaya Mint Smoothie

Papaya Carrot Pineapple Smoothie

Quatro Lamponi Mirtillo Negress Ribes Smoothie (4 Berries Smoothie)

Berries Kefir Smoothie

Red Currants Blueberry Smoothie

Cucumber Carrot Date Smoothie

Raspberry Sesame Smoothie

Yellow Tomato Passion Fruit Smoothie

Raspberry Cucumber Smoothie

Blackberry Kefir Smoothie

Cantaloupe Raspberry red Currant Smoothie

Papaya Cauliflower Smoothie

Carrot Cucumber Smoothie

Cantaloupe Papaya Smoothie

Strawberry Chia Spinach Smoothie

Red Dragon Fruit (Pitaya) Smoothie

Blueberry Yogurt & Spinach Smoothie

Beet Apple Smoothie

Blueberry Avocado Smoothie

Beet & Beet Smoothie

Chokecherry Cauliflower Smoothie

Purple Beet Smoothie

Purple Cabbage smoothie

Purple Cauliflower Smoothie

Acai Strawberries Smoothie

Red Grapefruit & Beets Smoothie

Purple Carrots Smoothie

Blueberry Banana Smoothie

Beet Kale Smoothie

Purple Kale Smoothie

Purple Endive & Fig Smoothie

Purple Queen Smoothie

Black Smoothie

Blueberry Kefir & Spinach Smoothie

Blackberry Yogurt & Purple Carrots Smoothie

Blackberry, Purple Kale and Mint Smoothie

Blackberry Banana Smoothie

Blueberry & Coconut Smoothie

Blueberry, Coconut Flakes & Sesame Seeds Smoothie

Blueberry & Purple Cauliflower Smoothie

Blueberry & Kefir Smoothie

Blueberry & Almond Smoothie

Smoothies Introduction

Hello,

My name is Don Orwell, and my blog SuperfoodsToday.com is dedicated to Superfoods lifestyle. I was able to lose 80 pounds in 2009 and keep them off by eating only regular everyday Superfoods. After several Superfoods related books, I decided to write one about smoothies. I hope you will enjoy the recipes I prepared for you.

Recipes text has only ingredients listed. Instructions for making a perfect smoothie are given below:

Put the liquid in first. Surrounded by tea or yogurt, the blender blades can move freely. Next, add chunks of fruits or vegetables. Leafy greens are going into the pitcher last. Preferred liquid is green tea, but you can use almond or coconut milk or herbal tea.

Start slow. If your blender has speeds, start it on low to break up big pieces of fruit. Continue blending until you get a puree. If your blender can pulse, pulse a few times before switching to a puree mode. Once you have your liquid and fruit pureed, start adding greens, very slowly. Wait until previous batch of greens has been completely blended. I use Vitamix blenders because they're sturdy and offer 7 year warranty. That was definitely the best investment in my health.

Thicken? Added too much tea or coconut milk? Thicken your smoothie by adding ice cubes, flax meal, chia seeds or oatmeal. Once you get used to various tastes of smoothies, add any seaweed, spirulina, chlorella powder or ginger for additional kick. Experiment with any Superfoods in powder form at this point. Think of adding any nut butter or sesame paste too or some

Superfoods oils.

Rotate! Rotate your greens; don't always drink the same smoothie! At the beginning try 2 different greens every week and later introduce third and fourth one weekly. And keep rotating them. Don't use spinach and kale all the time. Try beets greens, they have a pinch of pink in them and that add great color to your smoothie. Here is the list of leafy green for you to try: spinach, kale, dandelion, chards, beet leaves, arugula, lettuce, collard greens, bok choy, cabbage, cilantro, parsley.

Flavor! Flavor smoothies with ground vanilla bean, cinnamon, raw honey, nutmeg, cloves, almond butter, cayenne pepper, ginger or just about any seeds or chopped nuts combination.

Not only are green smoothies high in nutrients, vitamins and fiber, they can also make any vegetable you probably don't like (be it kale, spinach or broccoli) taste great. The secret behind blending the perfect smoothie is using sweet fruits or nuts or seeds to give your drink a unique taste.

There's a reason kale and spinach seem to be the main ingredients in almost every green smoothie. Not only do they give smoothies their verdant color, they are also packed with calcium, protein and iron.

Although blending alone increases the accessibility of carotenoids, since the presence of fats is known to increase carotenoid absorption from leafy greens, it is possible that coconut oil, nuts and seeds in a smoothie could increase absorption further.

Fruits and Veggies preparation

• Wash fruits and veggies

• Pluck leaves and stems from berries

• Core apples (optional)

• Peel orange, lemon, lime, grapefruit, kiwi, beet, pomegranate, ginger, dragon fruit and banana

• Peel and take the seeds out of papaya

• Remove seeds from peppers, apricots, peaches, cherries, plums and prunes

• Mangos, melons and avocados should be peeled, and inner seed taken out

• Watermelons should have their outer rind removed.

• Scoop out the flesh from passion fruit

• Cut fruits and veggies in 2-inch slices

RED SMOOTHIES

Carrot Date Smoothie

2 Carrots

2 Apples

1 cup of crushed ice

Pinch of nutmeg

½ tsp. Cinnamon

1 tbsp. Minced ginger

2 dates

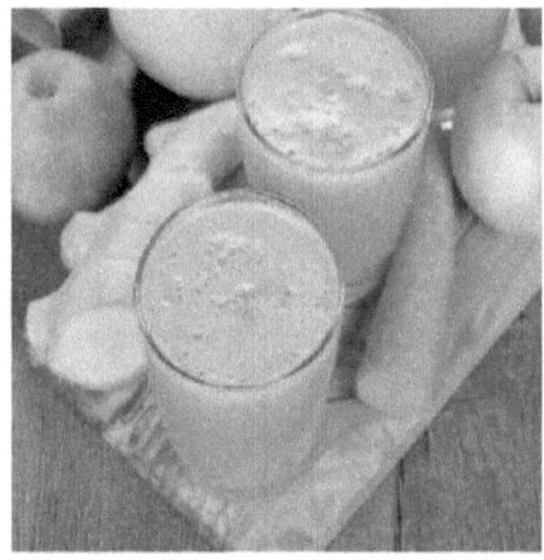

Spinach Berries Smoothie

- ½ cup almond milk
- ½ cup water
- 1 carrot
- 1 cup spinach
- 1 cup frozen raspberries
- 1 tablespoon Chia seeds
- 1 tablespoon fresh mint
- ½ teaspoon raw honey

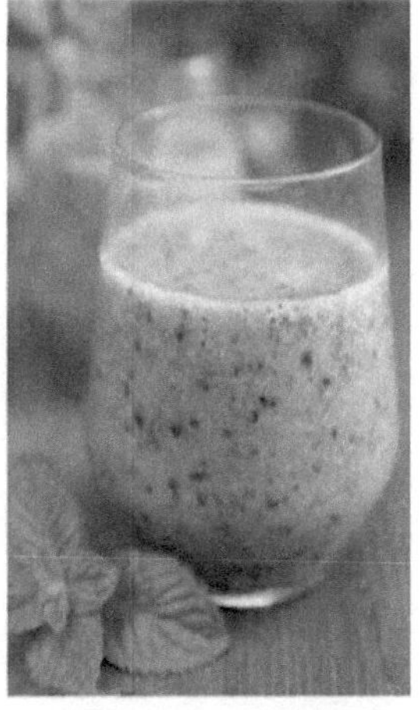

Watermelon Apple smoothie

- 1 cup Seedless Watermelon

- ½ cup Pomegranate

- 2 apples

- 1/2 cup Raspberries

- 1 tbsp. Maqui

- 1 cup Yerba Mate tea

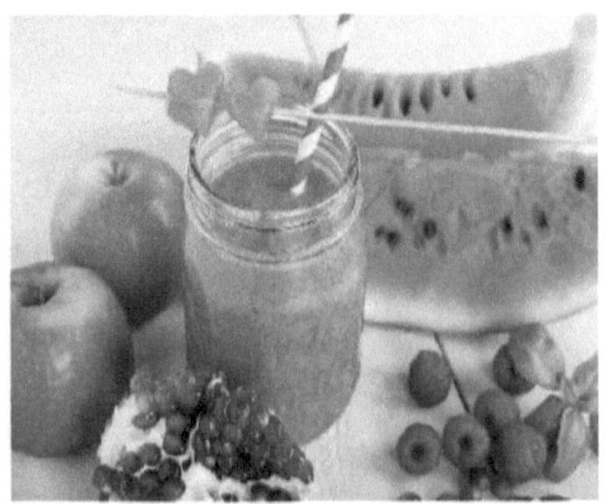

Watermelon Red Grapefruit Smoothie

- 1 cup seedless Watermelon

- 1 Red Grapefruit

- 1 cup red spinach

- 1 cup crushed ice

- 2 tablespoons ground flax seeds

- 1 tbsp. Bee Pollen

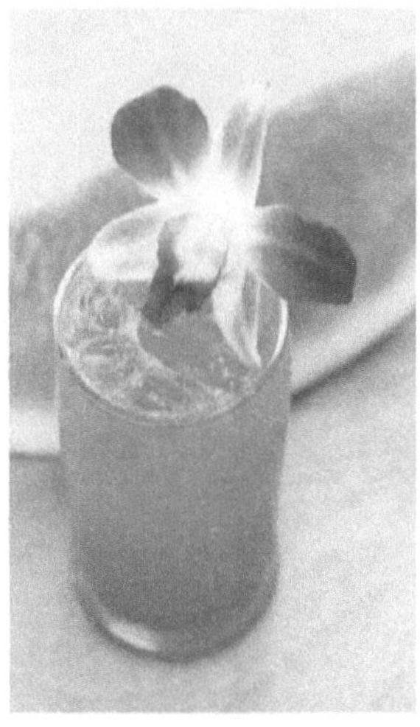

Strawberry Carrot Smoothie

- 1 cup frozen strawberries

- 1 banana

- 1 carrot

- 1 cup crushed ice

- 2 tablespoons Hemp seeds

- 1 tsp. Fresh Mint

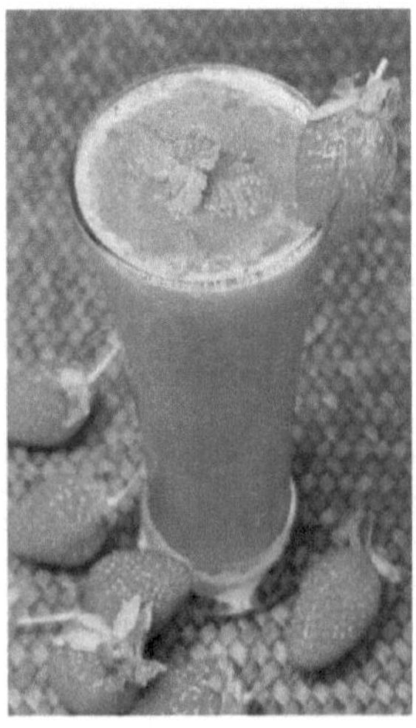

Red Peppers Tomato Salad Smoothie

1 cup Red Peppers

1/2 medium avocado

2 medium tomatoes

1 cucumber

2 tablespoons lemon juice

1 tsp. olive oil & 1 tsp. chopped garlic

Pinch of sea salt & 1 tbsp. dill

1/2 cup crushed ice

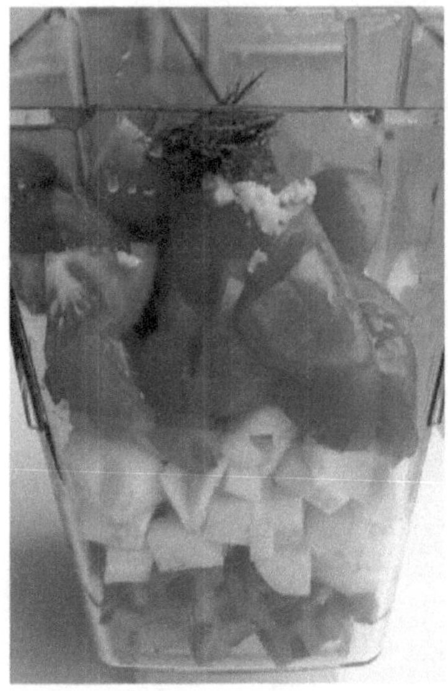

Apricots & Carrots Smoothie

4 apricots

1 apple

1 cup red spinach

2 carrots

1 cup water

1 tbsp. Maca

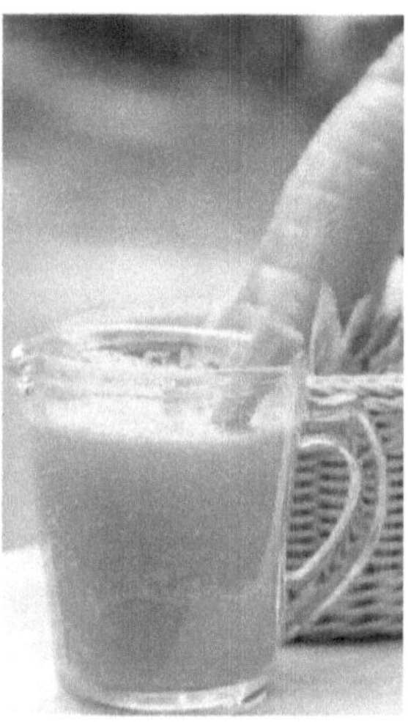

Watermelon Strawberries Smoothie

- 1 cup seedless watermelon, cubed
- ½ cup strawberries
- ½ cup low-fat plain yogurt
- 3 ice cubes
- 1 tbsp. Ground coconut
- 1 tbsp. Acai

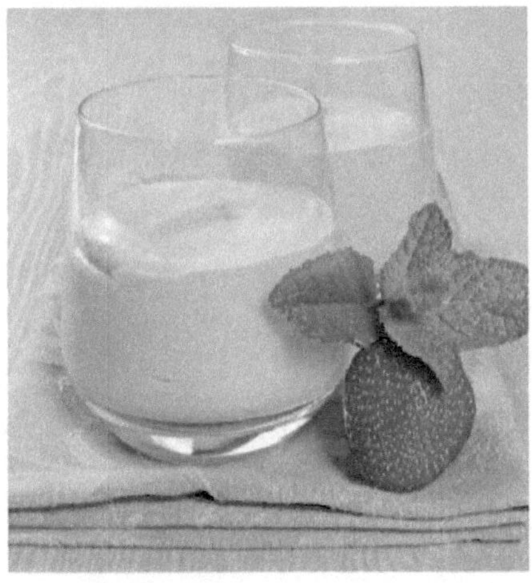

Red Swiss Smoothie

- 1 cup Red Swiss chard
- ½ cup raspberries, frozen
- ½ cup peaches, frozen
- ½ cup pineapple, frozen
- 1 tbsp. Pumpkin seeds
- 1 orange
- 1 cup crushed ice

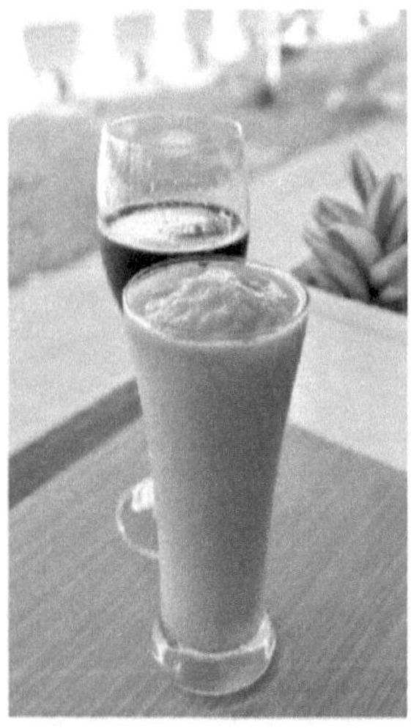

Red Leaf Lettuce Smoothie

- 1 cup Red Leaf Lettuce

- 1 Bananas

- 1 Celery stalk

- 1/2 cup Strawberry

- 1/2 cup Raspberry

- 1 cup crushed ice

- 1 clove & pinch of nutmeg

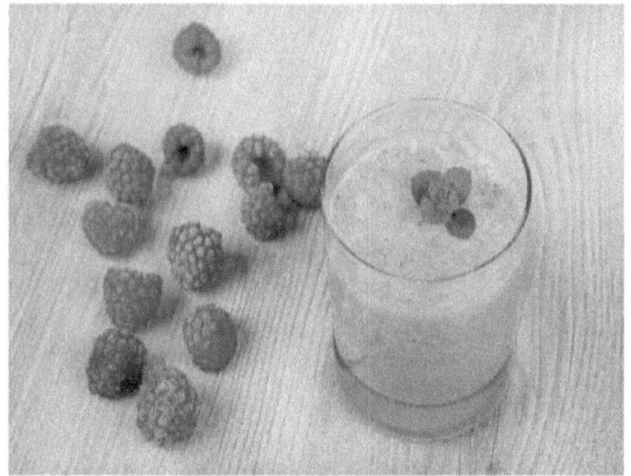

Red Veggie Smoothie

- 1 cup chopped tomato

- 1 kiwi

- 1 banana

- 1/2 celery stalk

- 1/4 cup each cilantro and spinach

- 1 tbsp. Olive oil

- Pinch of sea salt

- 1/2 cup ice

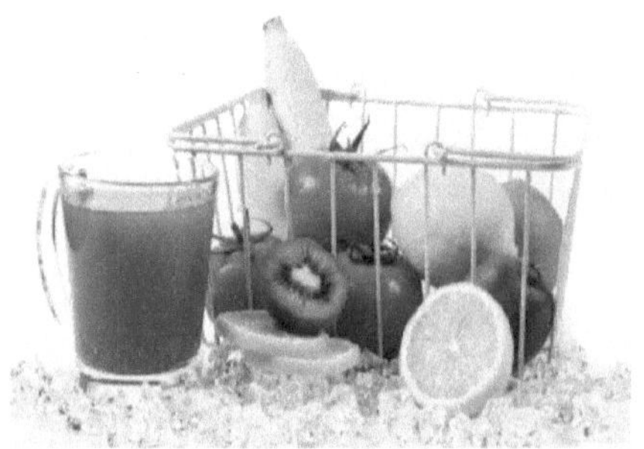

Papaya Diva Smoothie

- 1 cup Red Endive

- 1 cup chopped Papaya

- 1 banana

- 1 tbsp. chopped fresh Ginger

- 1 cup crushed ice

- 1 tbsp. Cashew butter

- Top with Goji berries

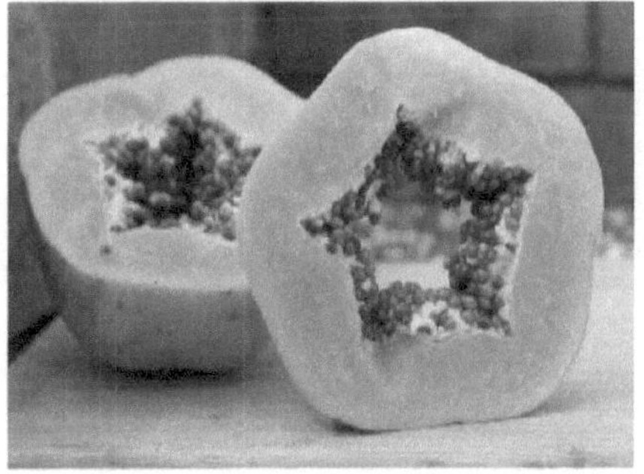

Tomato Onion Smoothie

- 2 Tomatoes

- 1/2 Cucumber

- ¼ cup Cilantro

- 1/2 of small onion

- 1 tbsp. Olive oil

- 1 cup crushed ice

- Juice of 1/2 lime

- 1 Avocado

- Pinch of sea salt

- 1 tbsp. Fresh Basil

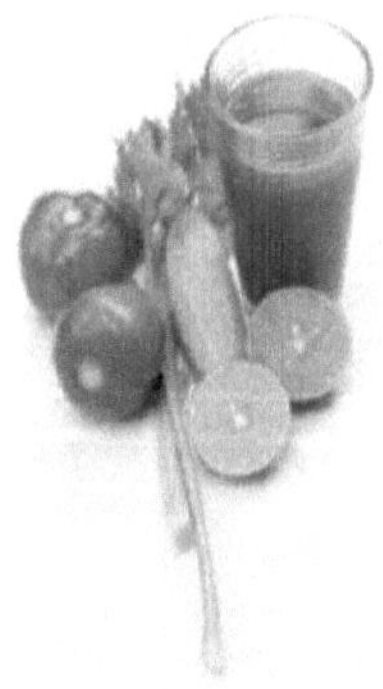

Pomegranates & Berries smoothie

- 1 cup Cherries

- ½ cup Raspberries

- 1 cup Pomegranates

- ½ cup Strawberries

- 1 cup Yerba Mate tea

- 1 tbsp. Chlorella

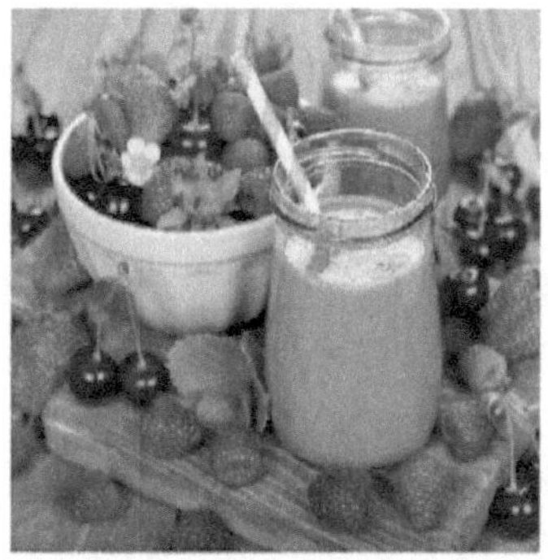

Swiss Peach Smoothie

• 1 cup Red Swiss chard

• ½ cup raspberries, frozen

• 1 cup peaches, frozen

• 1 blood orange

• 1 cup crushed ice

• 1 tbsp. Maca

• 1 tbsp. Coconut flakes on top

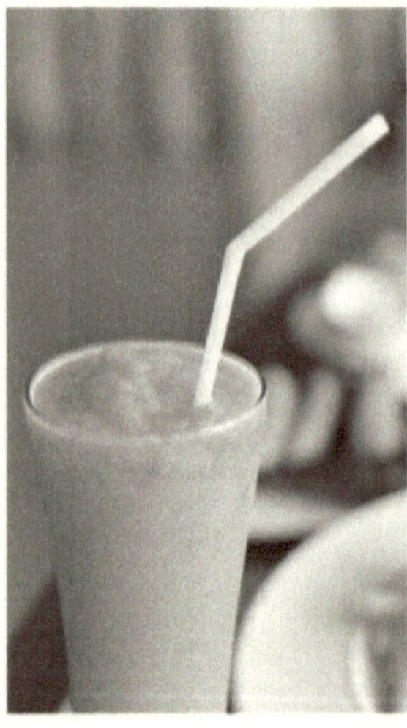

Red Avocado Carrot Smoothie

- 2 carrots

- 1 banana

- ½ avocado

- 2 apple

- Juice of ½ lemon

- 1 cup crushed ice

- 1 tsp. ginger

- Top with Bee Pollen

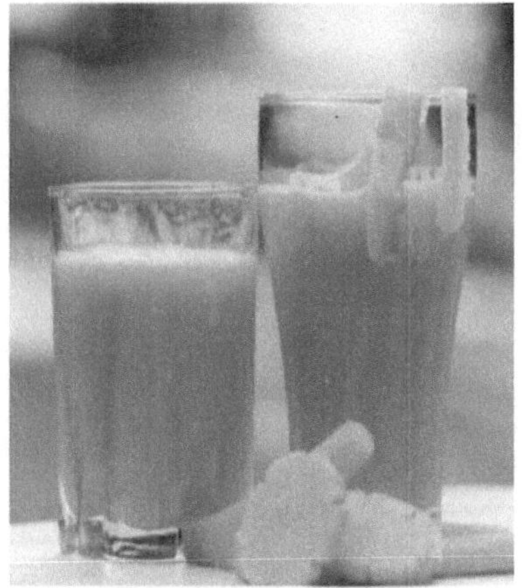

Radicchio Cranberry Smoothie

- 1 cup fresh Cranberries
- 1 apple
- ½ cup Red Spinach
- ½ Avocado
- 1/2 cup chopped Radicchio
- 1 tbsp. Acai
- 1 cup crushed ice

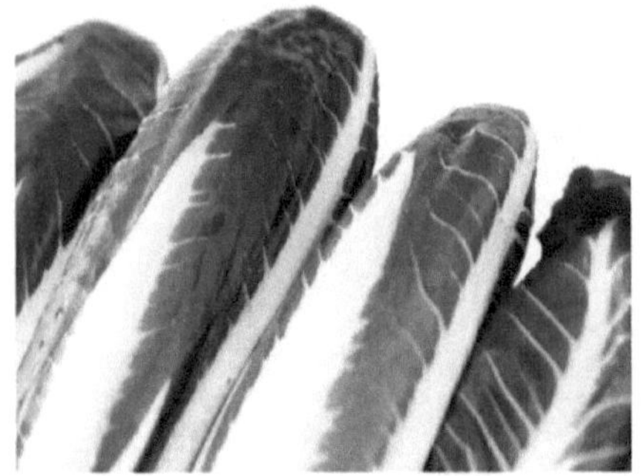

Red Currants Pumpkin Smoothie

- 1 cup pumpkin puree

- 1 cup red currants

- 1 cup ginger tea

- 1 tbsp. raw honey

- 1 clove

- Pinch of nutmeg

- Pinch of cinnamon

- 1 tbsp. Chia Seeds

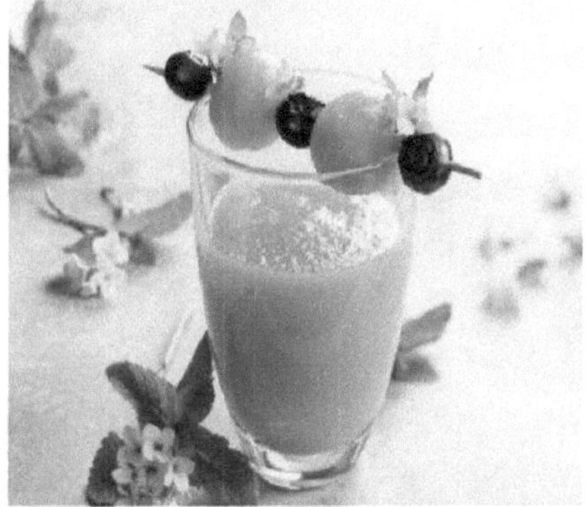

Cucumber Beet Smoothie

- 1 Large Beet
- ½ Cucumber
- 1 Apple
- 1 clove garlic
- 1 tbsp. Minced ginger
- 1 cup crushed ice
- 1 tbsp. Crushed Seaweed (Wakame or Arame)

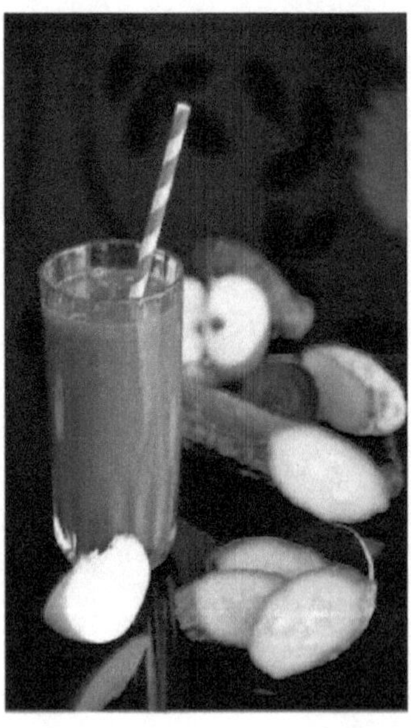

Rhubarb Avocado Smoothie

- 1 cup chopped Rhubarb

- 1/2 Avocado

- 1 cup hibiscus tea

- 1 tbsp. Cacao nibs

- 1 tbsp. Chopped pecans

- 2 tbsp. Sesame seeds sprinkled

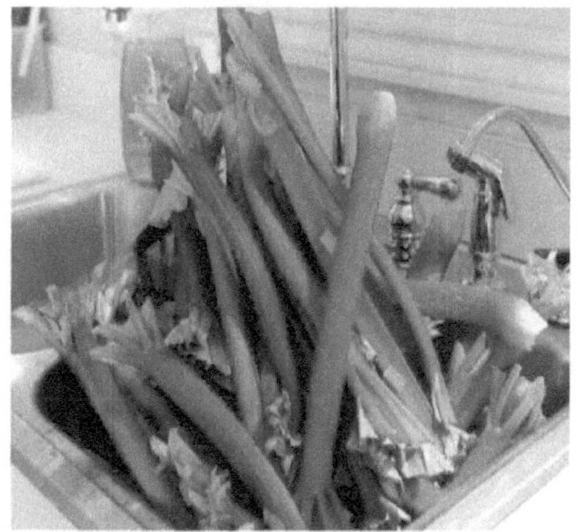

Blood Orange Smoothie

- 2 Blood Oranges

- 2 carrots

- 1 cup Raspberries

- 1 cup hibiscus tea

- 1 tbsp. Walnuts

- 2 tbsp. Ground <u>flax</u> seeds

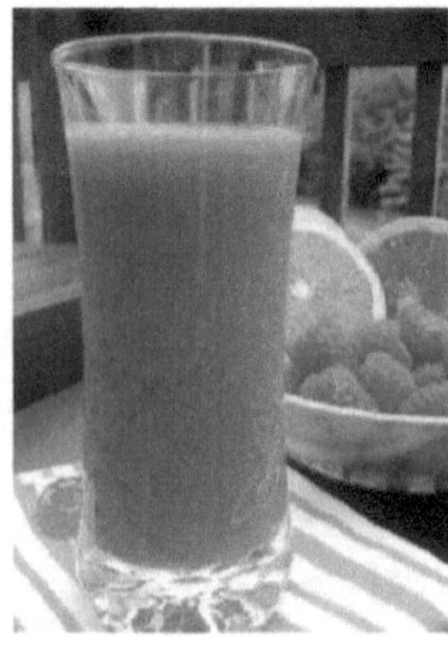

Papaya Red Spinach Smoothie

- 1 cup chopped Papaya

- 1 banana

- 1 cup red spinach

- 1 cup crushed ice

- 1 tablespoon Maca

- Top with 1 tablespoon dried chokecherries

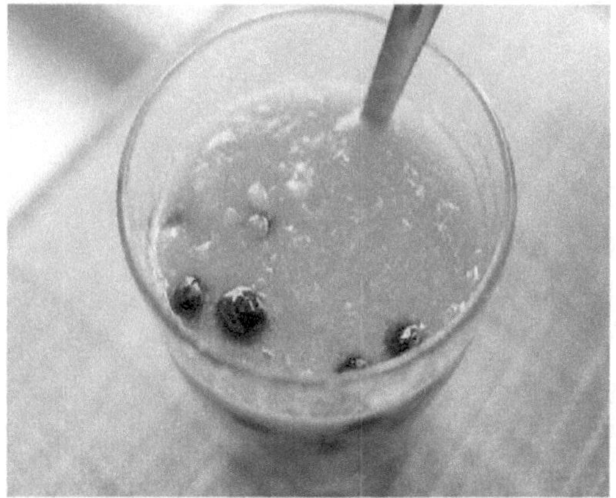

Red Grapefruit Smoothie

- 1 large red Grapefruit

- 1 cup Red Endive

- 1 cup crushed ice

- 2 tbsp. Sunflower seeds butter

- 1 tbsp. <u>Hemp</u> seeds sprinkled

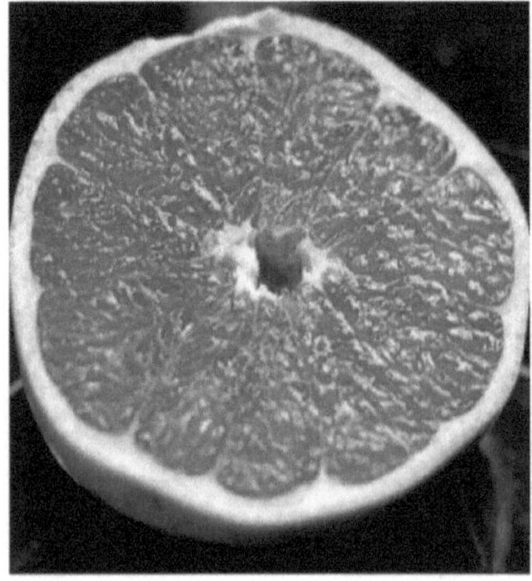

Raspberry Red Lettuce Smoothie

- 1 cup Red Leaf Lettuce

- 1 cup frozen Raspberries

- 2 Red Apples

- 1 tbsp. Goji berries

- 1 cup white tea

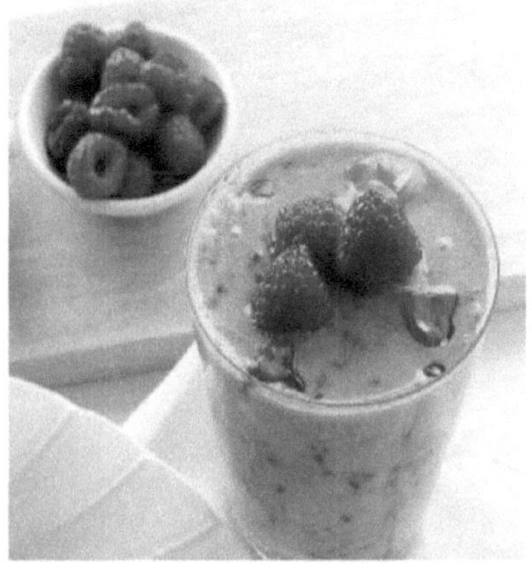

Cranberry Red Leaf Lettuce Smoothie

- 1 cups Red Leaf Lettuce

- 1 Banana

- 1 tbsp. Tahini

- 1 cup fresh Cranberries

- 1 cup crushed ice

- Top with Coconut flakes

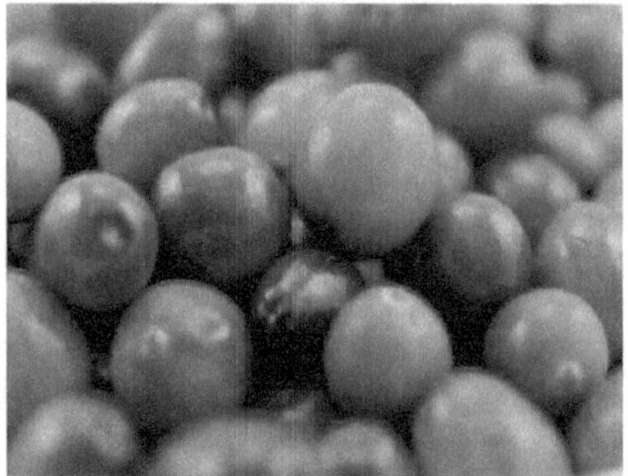

50 Shades of Smoothies

Green Layer: 2 Kiwis + 1 cup spinach + 2 ice cubes

Yellow Layer: 1 Mango + 1 Peach + 2 ice cubes

Red Layer: 1 cup of Strawberries + 1 cup of Raspberries

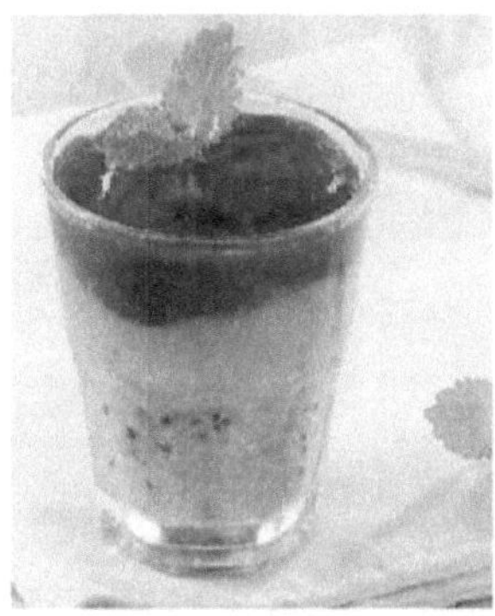

Frozen Berries Smoothie

1 cup frozen raspberries

1 cup frozen blueberries

1 cup of kefir

Pinch of nutmeg

1 tbsp. Minced ginger

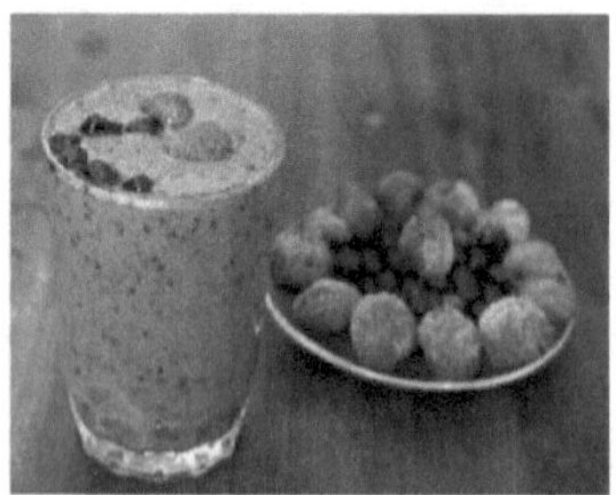

Superfoods Smoothie Popsicles

Green Layer: 2 Kiwis + 1 Granny Smith apple + 1 ice cube

Yellow Layer: 1 Mango + 1 Orange + 1 ice cube

Red Layer: 1 cup of seedless watermelon + 1/2 cup of Raspberries

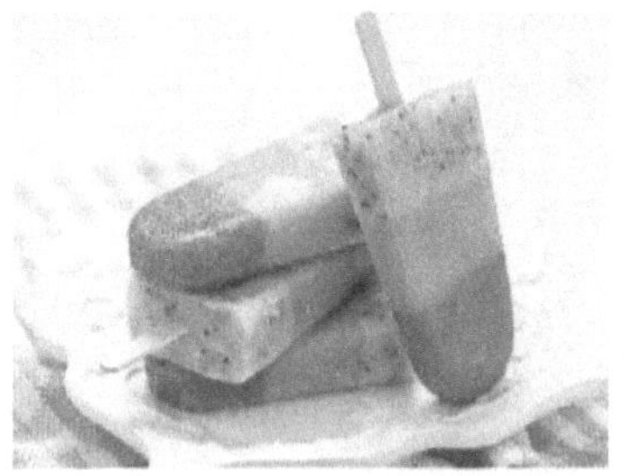

Pomegranate Watermelon Smoothie

1 cup seedless watermelon

1 cup Pomegranate seeds

1 cup of crushed ice

2 carrots

½ tsp. Mint

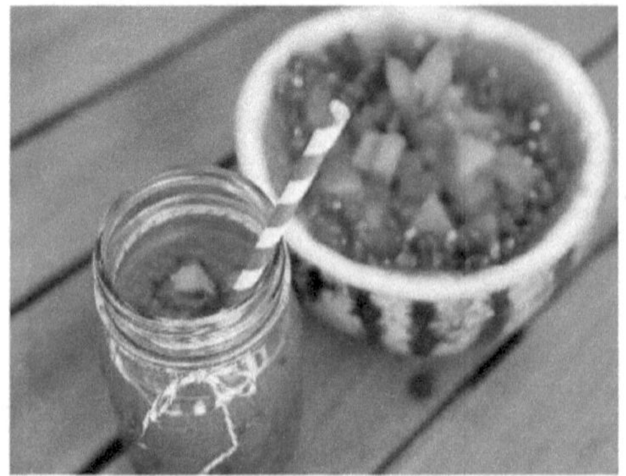

Orange Carrot Smoothie

2 Carrots

2 Oranges

1 cup of crushed ice

Pinch of cinnamon

1 tbsp. Minced ginger

1 tbsp. Chia seeds

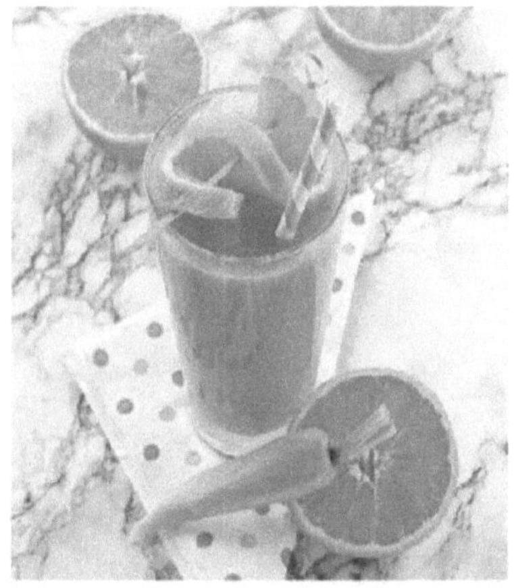

Carrot Orange Papaya Smoothie

2 Carrots

1 Papaya

1 Orange

1 cup of crushed ice

Pinch of nutmeg

½ tsp. Cinnamon

1 tsp. Bee Pollen

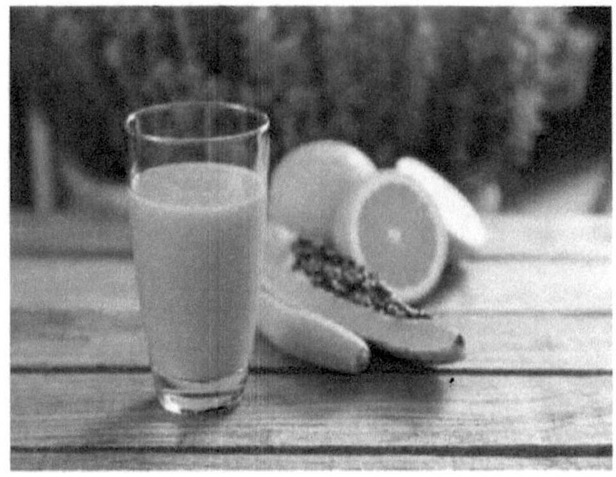

Carrot Pumpkin Smoothie

2 Carrots

2 cups of chopped pumpkin

1 cup of crushed ice

Pinch of nutmeg

½ tsp. Cinnamon

1 tbsp. Minced parsley

1 tsp. pumpkin seeds

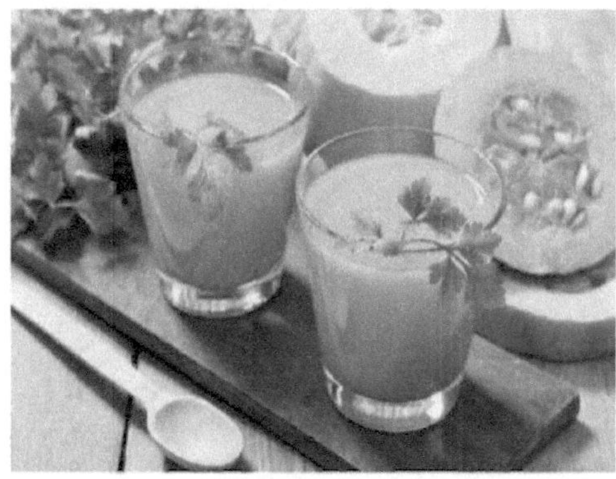

Raspberry Cauliflower Smoothie

2 Cups raspberries

1 cup cauliflower florets

1 cup of crushed ice

1 tsp. Acai

½ tsp. Maqui

1 tbsp. ground flax seeds

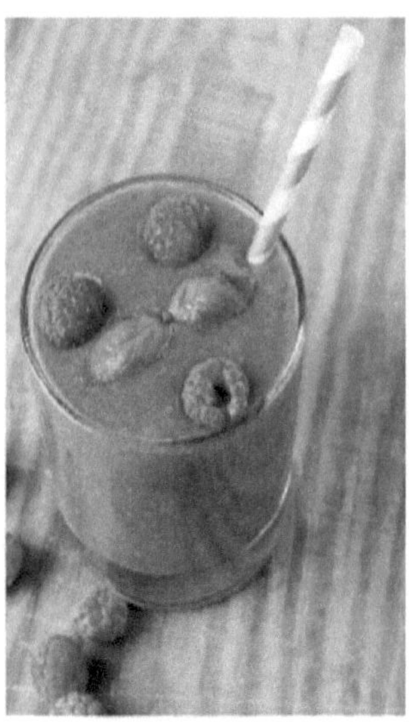

Pomegranate Yogurt Smoothie

1 cup Pomegranate seeds

2 ice cubes

1 cup of low fat yogurt

½ tsp. Bee Pollen

1 tbsp. sunflower seeds

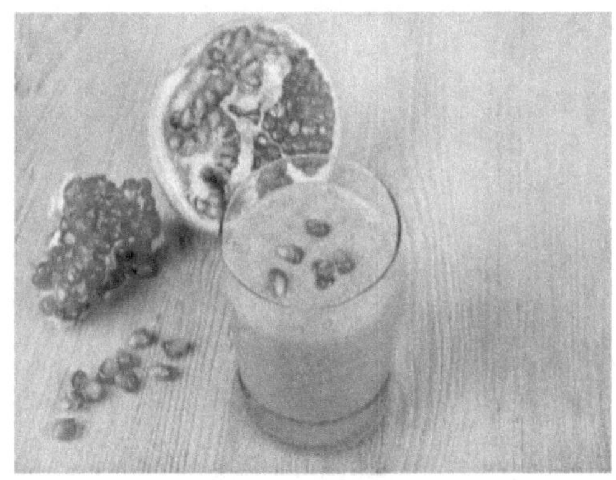

Mango Papaya Mint Smoothie

1 chopped Mango

1 chopped Papaya

1 cup of crushed ice

Pinch of nutmeg

½ tsp. Mint

1 tbsp. Papaya Seeds

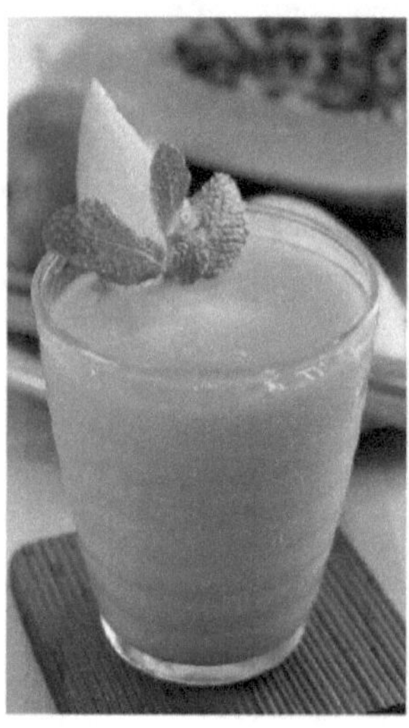

Papaya Carrot Pineapple Smoothie

2 Carrots

1 cup pineapple chunks

1 cup of crushed ice

1 cup od chopped Papaya

½ tsp. Cinnamon

1 tbsp. Minced ginger

1 tbsp. Papaya seeds

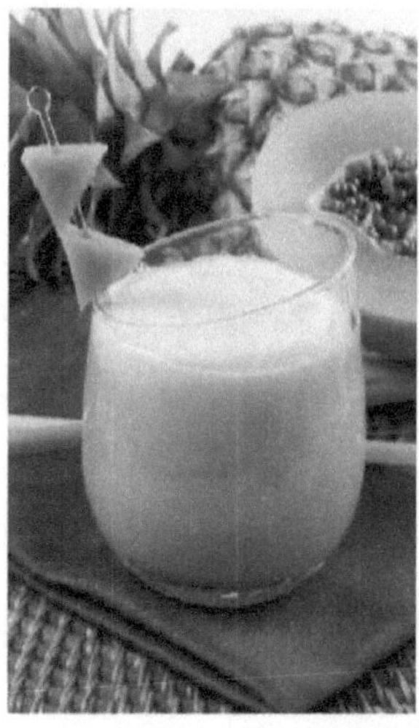

Quatro Lamponi Mirtillo Negress Ribes Smoothie (4 Berries Smoothie)

½ cup raspberries

½ cup blueberries

½ cup blackberries

½ cup red currants

1 cup of crushed ice

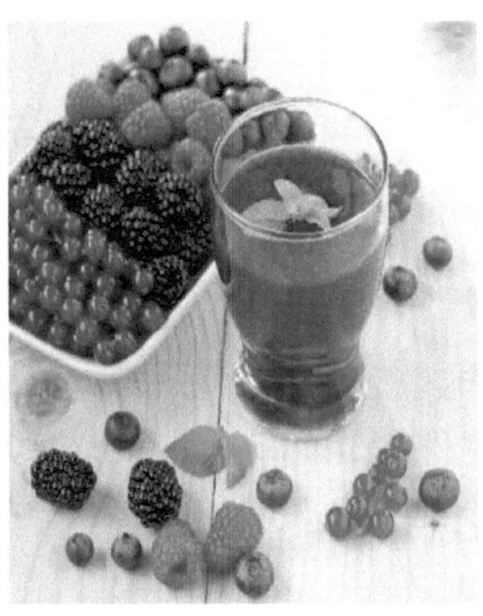

Berries Kefir Smoothie

1/2 cup blackberries

½ cup raspberries

1/2 cup of crushed ice

1 cup Kefir

1 tbsp. Chia seeds

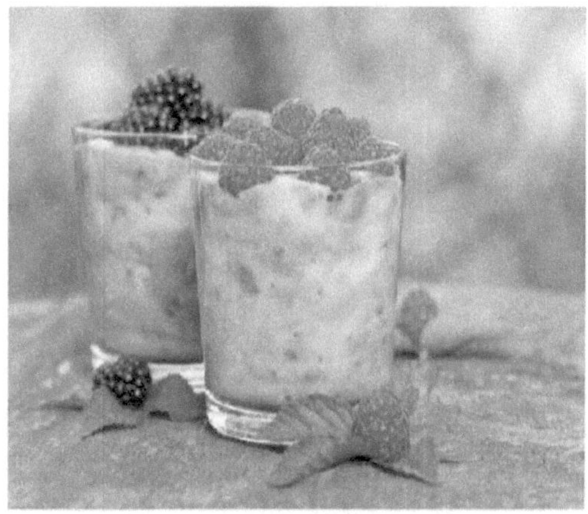

Red Currants Blueberry Smoothie

1 cup Red Spinach

1/2 cup blueberries

1/2 cup red currants

1 cup of crushed ice

Pinch of nutmeg

½ tsp. sesame seeds

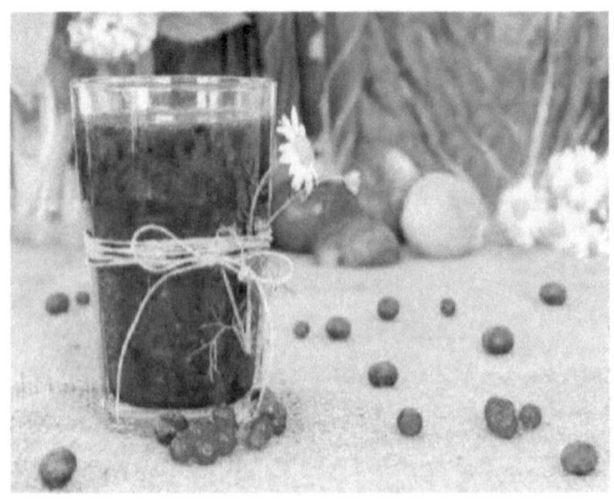

Cucumber Carrot Date Smoothie

2 Carrots

2 Cucumbers

1/2 cup of crushed ice

½ tsp. Cinnamon

1 tbsp. Minced ginger

2 dates

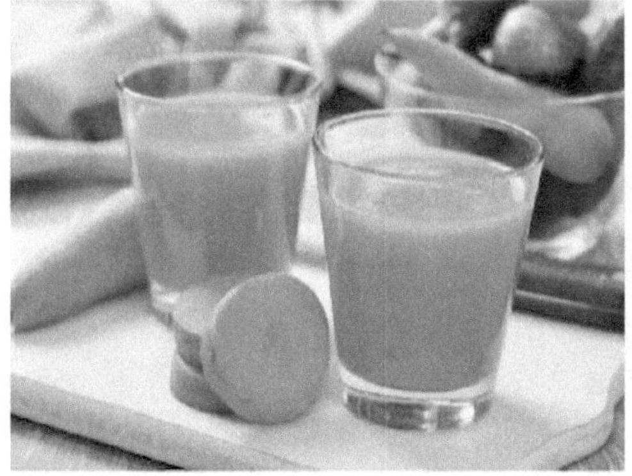

Raspberry Sesame Smoothie

2 cups raspberries

2 Tbsp. tahini

1 cup of crushed ice

1 tbsp. Sesame seeds

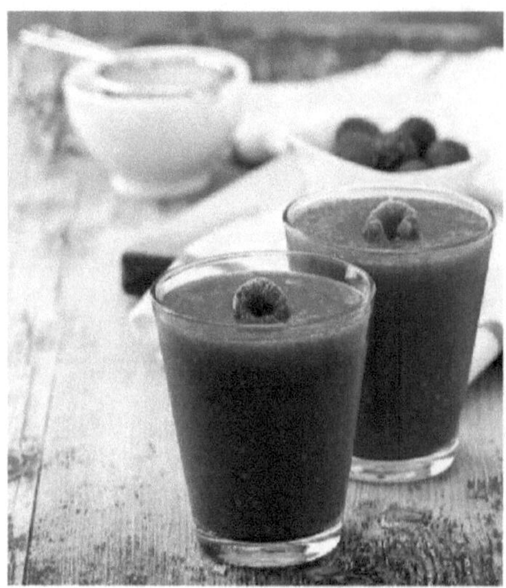

Yellow Tomato Passion Fruit Smoothie

2 yellow tomatoes

1 yellow pepper

1 cup of crushed ice

2 oranges

1 chopped passion fruit

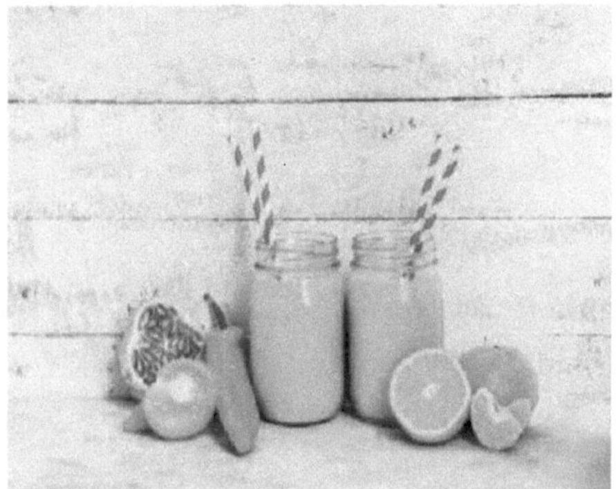

Raspberry Cucumber Smoothie

1 cucumber

2 cups raspberries

1 cup of crushed ice

1 tbsp. Minced ginger

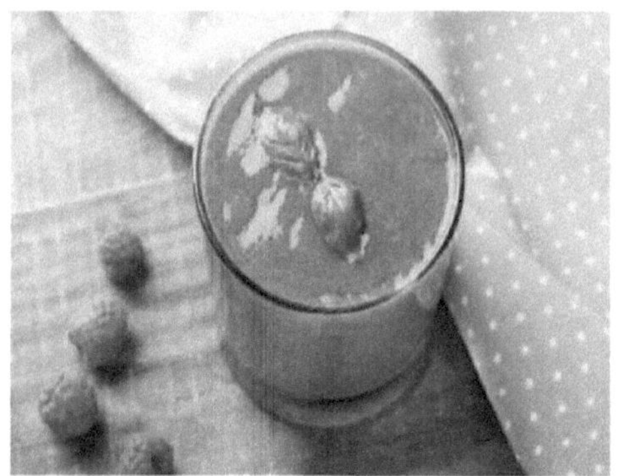

Blackberry Kefir Smoothie

1 cup Blackberries

1 cup Kefir

1 cup of crushed ice

½ tsp. mint leaves

2 lemon wedges for decoration

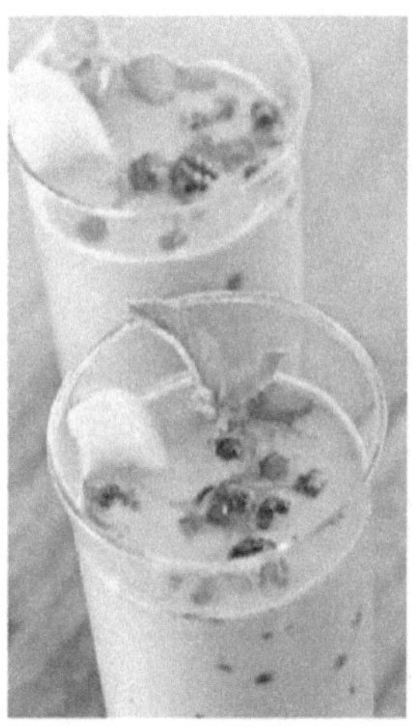

Cantaloupe Raspberry red Currant Smoothie

1 cup chopped cantaloupe

1 cup raspberries

1/2 red currants

1 cup of crushed ice

Pinch of nutmeg

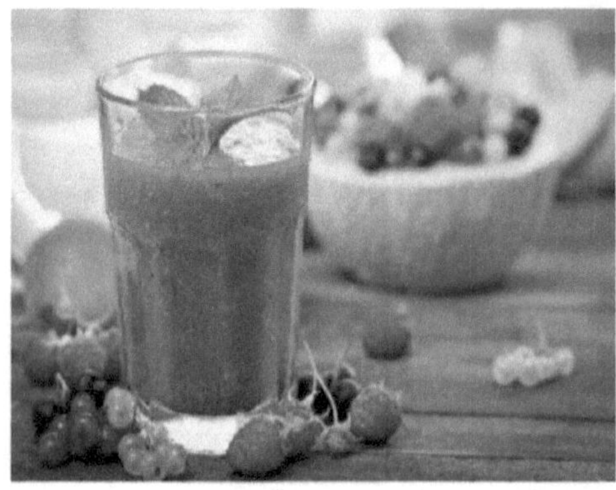

Papaya Cauliflower Smoothie

1 chopped Papaya

1 cup cauliflower florets

1 cup of crushed ice

Pinch of nutmeg

1 Tbsp. Lucuma powder

1 tbsp. Minced ginger

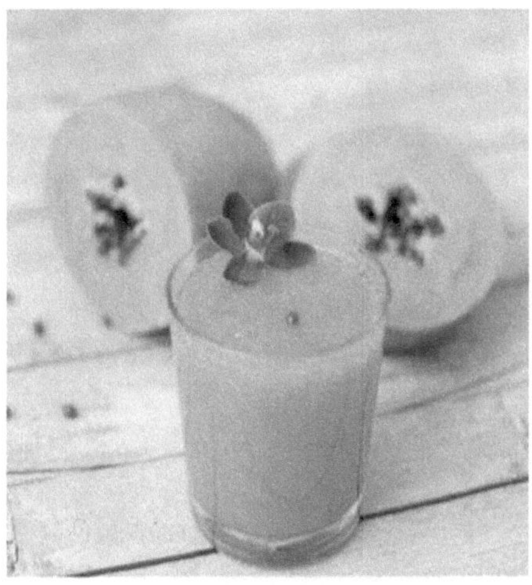

Carrot Cucumber Smoothie

2 Carrots

1 Apple

1 cup of crushed ice

2 Cucumbers

1 tbsp. Minced ginger

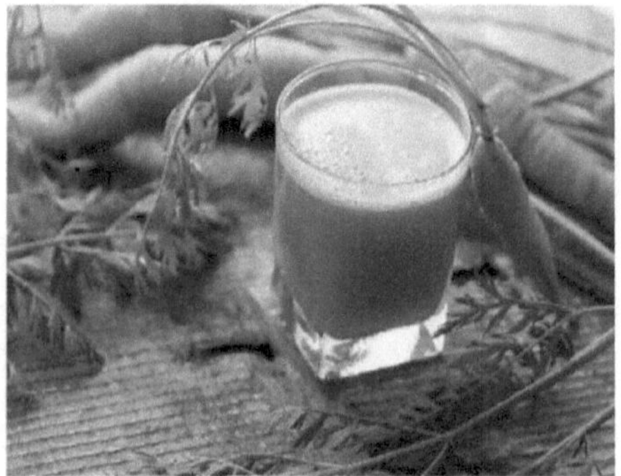

Pumpkin Date Smoothie

2 Carrots

1 cup chopped pumpkin

1 cup of crushed ice

Pinch of nutmeg

½ tsp. Cinnamon

1 tbsp. Minced ginger

2 dates

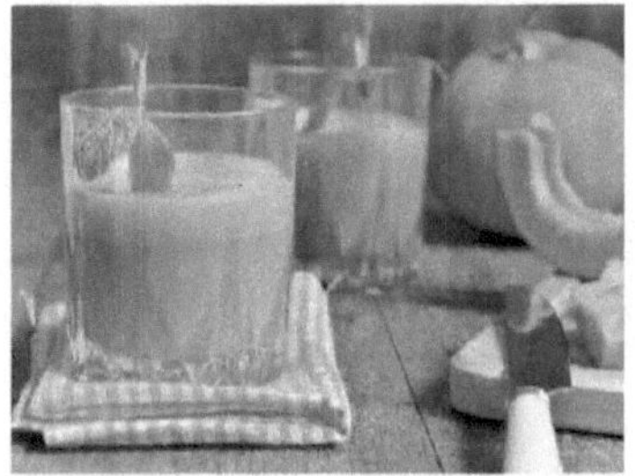

Pumpkin Kefir Smoothie

1 cup chopped pumpkin

1 Apple

1 cup of crushed ice

Pinch of nutmeg

½ tsp. Cinnamon

Pumpkin smoothie top with Kefir and Pumpkin seeds

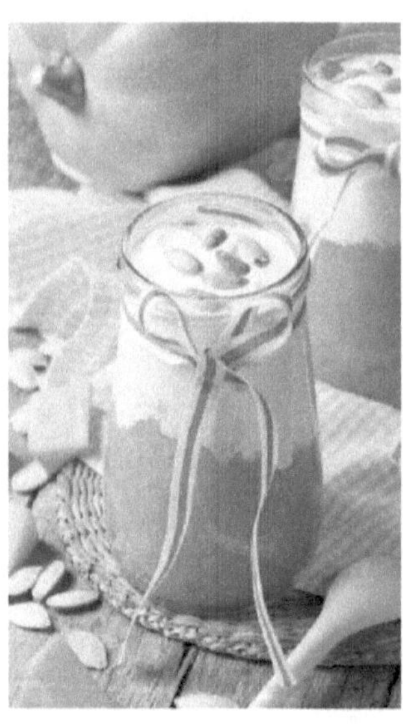

Cantaloupe Papaya Smoothie

1 chopped Papaya

1 cup chopped cantaloupe

1 banana

Juice from 1 lime

1 cup of crushed ice

1 tbsp. Minced ginger

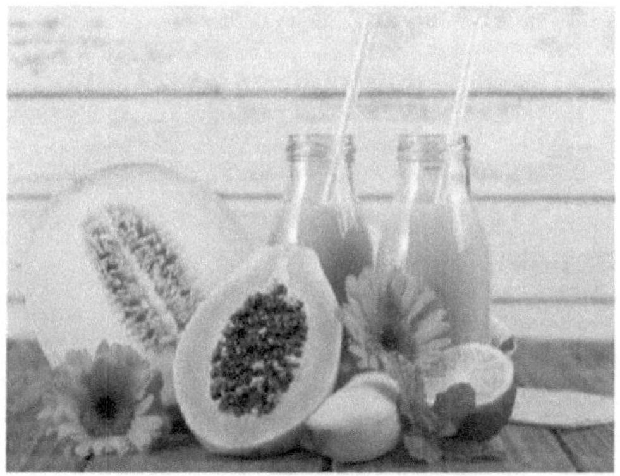

Buttermilk Cherry Banana Smoothie

1 cup buttermilk

1 cup frozen pitted cherries

1/2 cup of crushed ice

1 banana

½ cup of Strawberries

1 tbsp. Minced ginger

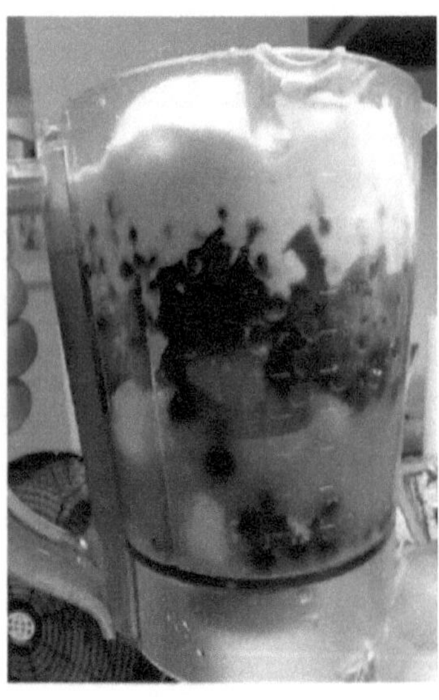

Strawberry Buttermilk Oats Smoothie

1 cup Strawberries

1/2 cup of crushed ice

1 cup buttermilk

2 tbsp. oats

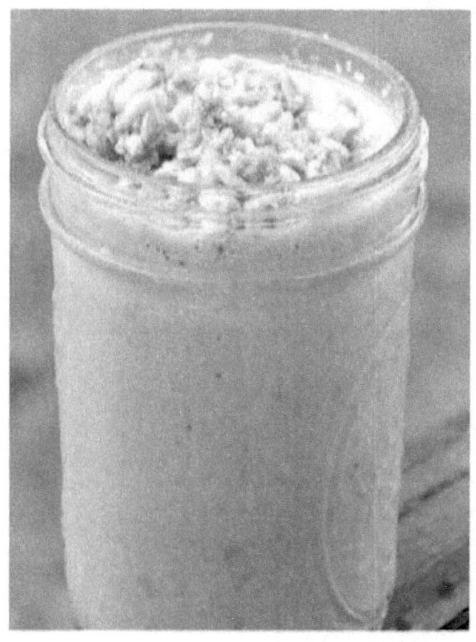

Strawberry Pineapple Bluebery Oats Smoothie

1 Cup Strawberries

1 banana

1 cup of crushed ice

Pinch of nutmeg

½ cup blueberries

½ cup pineapple chunks

3 tbsp. oats

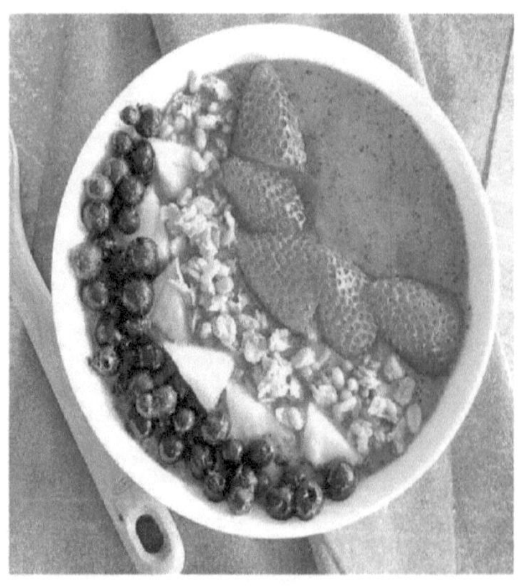

Strawberry Chia Spinach Smoothie

1 Cup Strawberries

1 cup spinach

1 banana

1 cup of crushed ice

2 Tbsp. Chia seeds

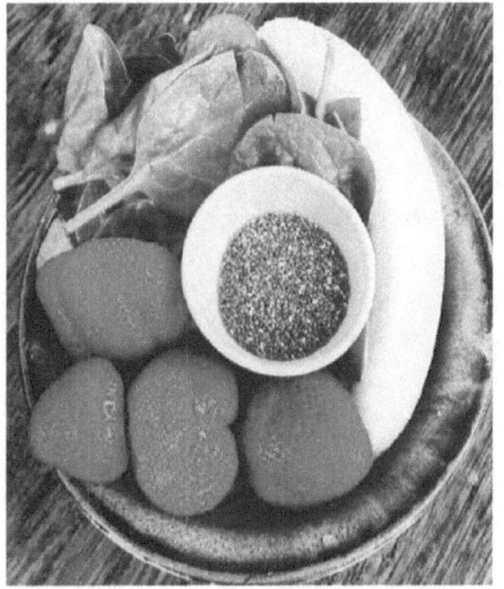

Red Dragon Fruit (Pitaya) Smoothie

- 2 purple carrots

- 2 tbsp. Almond Butter

- 1 cup Red Dragon fruit (Pitaya)

- 1 tbsp. Maca

- 1 Blood Orange

- 1 cup crushed ice

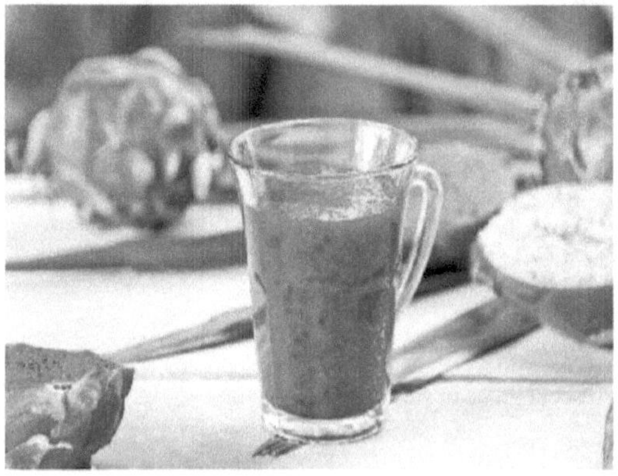

Blueberry Yogurt & Spinach Smoothie

- 1 cup blueberries

- 1 avocado

- 1 cup Red Chard

- 1 cup Yogurt

- 1/2 cup Mulberry

- 1 tbsp. Ground flax seeds

- ½ tsp. Cinnamon

- Top with Blueberries and Coconut flakes

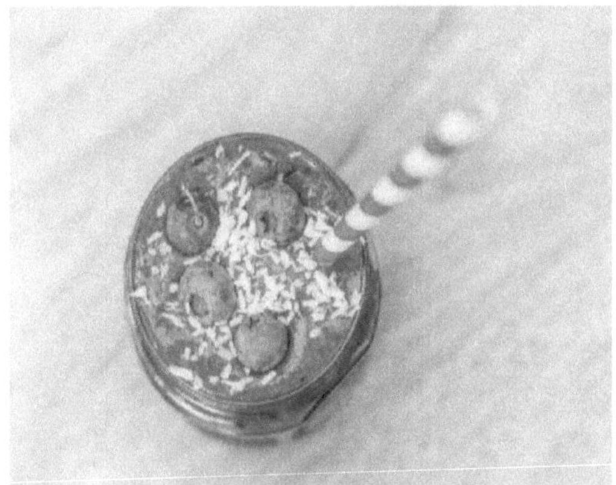

Beet Apple Smoothie
• 1 cup crushed ice

• 1/2 avocado, pitted

• 1 cup frozen strawberries

• 1 lemon, juiced

• 2 chopped celery stalks

• 1 large beet

• 1 apple

• 1 tablespoon coconut oil

• 1 tbsp. Acai

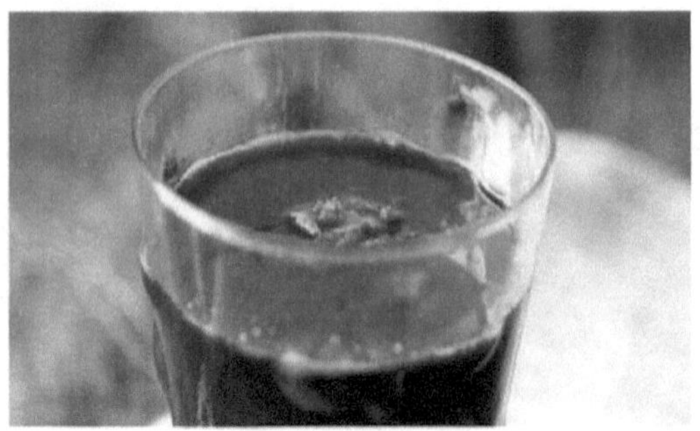

Blueberry Avocado Smoothie

- 1/2 avocado

- 1 cup spinach

- 1 cup blueberries, frozen

- 1 tsp. coconut oil

- 3/4 cup water

- 1 cup crushed ice

- Top with Cranberries

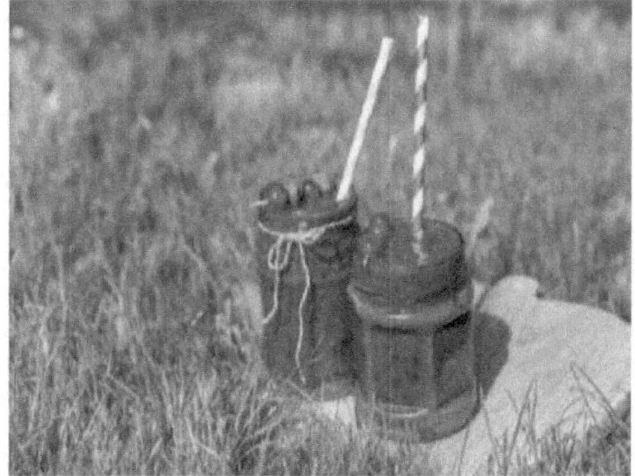

Beet & Beet Smoothie

- 2 cups Beet Greens

- 1 cup crushed ice

- 2 blood oranges,

- 1 large Beet

- Juice of ½ lemon

- 1 tbsp. Hemp seeds

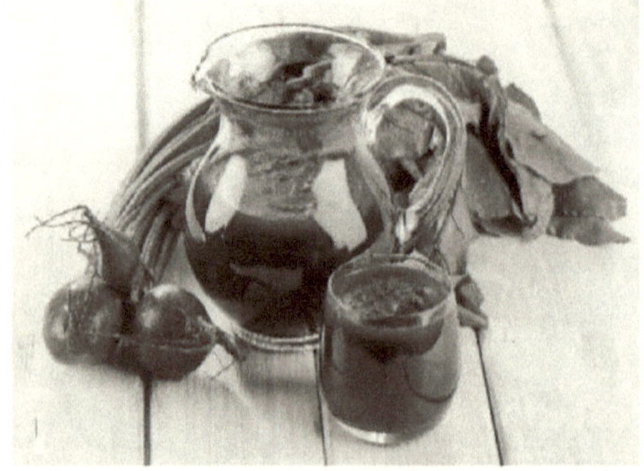

Chokecherry Cauliflower Smoothie

- 1 cup Chokecherries or 1/2 cup of dried Chokecherries

- ½ cup cauliflower

- 1 cup kefir

- 3 ice cubes

- 1 tbsp. Matcha

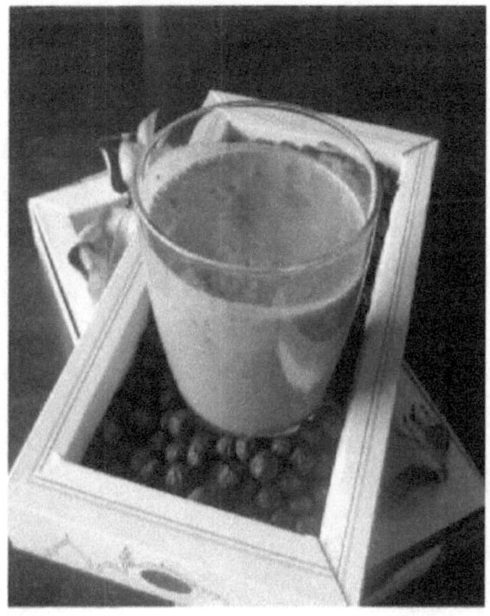

Purple Beet Smoothie

- 2 large beets
- ½ Avocado
- 1 cup Raspberry
- 1 tbsp. Chia seeds
- 1 carrot
- 1 cup crushed ice

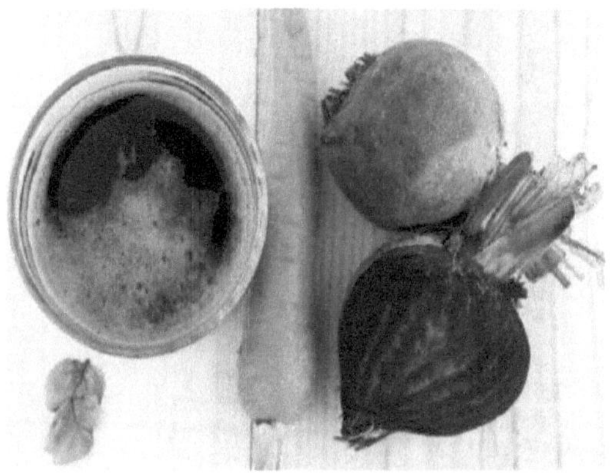

Purple Cabbage smoothie

- 1 cup Red Cabbage

- ½ Avocado

- 1 Kiwi

- 1 Banana

- 1 Brazil Nut

- 1 cup hibiscus tea

- 1 tbsp. Spirulina

- 1 cup crushed ice

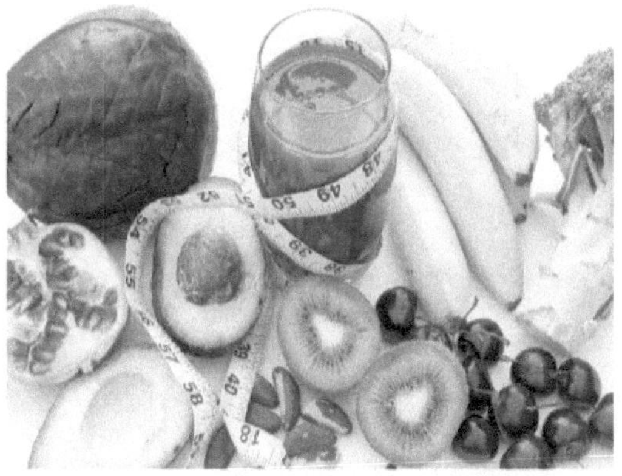

Purple Cauliflower Smoothie

• 1 cup Purple cauliflower

• 1 banana

• 1 cup Black Currants

• 1 tbsp. Chlorella

• 1 cup Chai tea

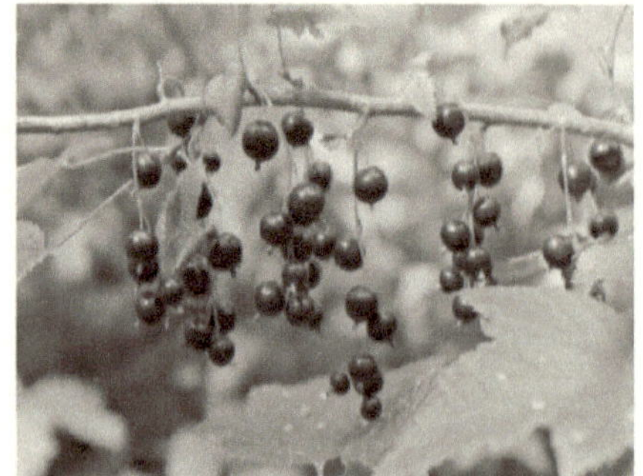

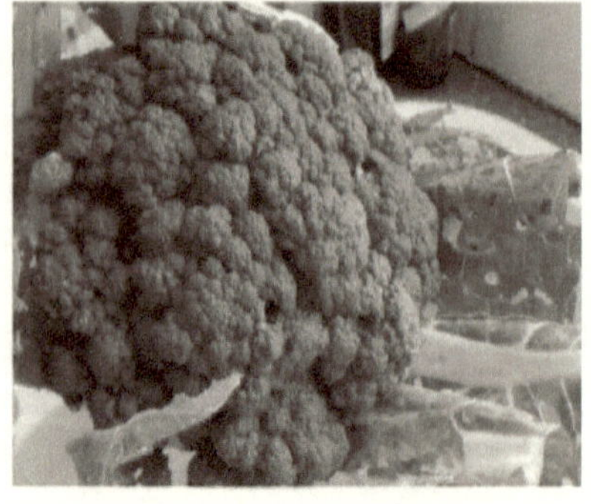

Acai Strawberries Smoothie

- 1 cup Acai berries or 1/4 cup of <u>Acai</u> powder

- ½ cup strawberries

- 1 cup low-fat plain yogurt

- 3 ice cubes

- 1 tbsp. <u>Bee Pollen</u>

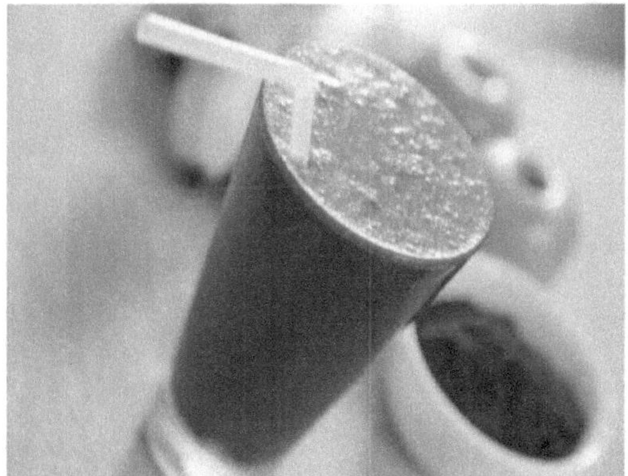

Red Grapefruit & Beets Smoothie

- 1 Red Grapefruit
- 1 large beet
- 1/2 cup frozen sliced peaches
- 1/2 cup frozen strawberries
- 1/2 cup frozen mango chunks
- 1 tbsp. Maca
- 1 cup crushed ice

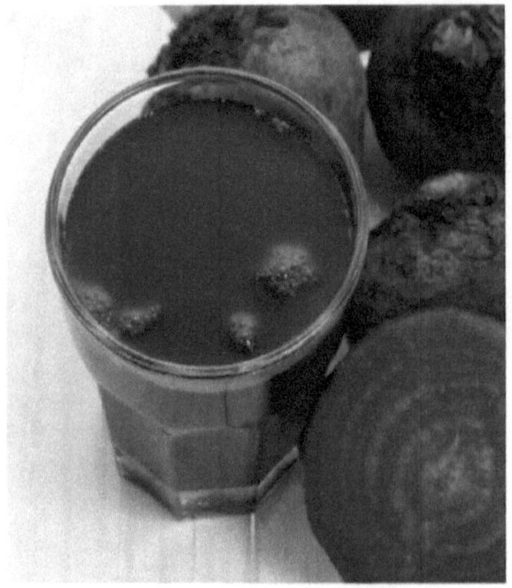

Purple Carrots Smoothie

- 3 purple carrots

- 2 tbsp. Almond Butter

- 1 cup Blackberries

- 1 tbsp. Chlorella

- 1 Orange

- 1 cup crushed ice

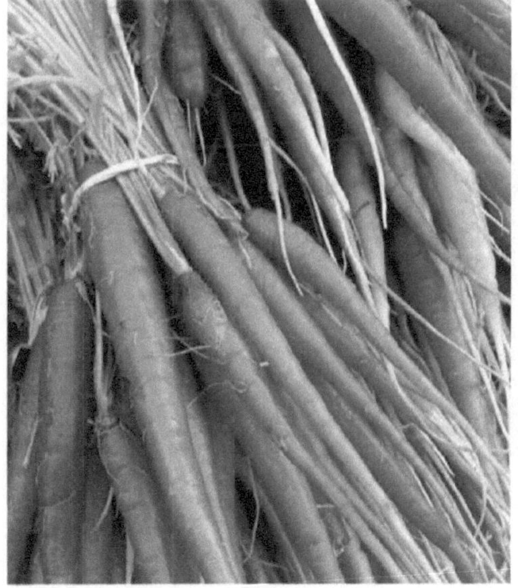

Blueberry Banana Smoothie

- 1 cup Blueberries

- 1 apple

- 1 banana

- 1 cup Red endive

- ½ cup crushed ice

- ½ cup water

- Top with Goji berries and shredded coconut

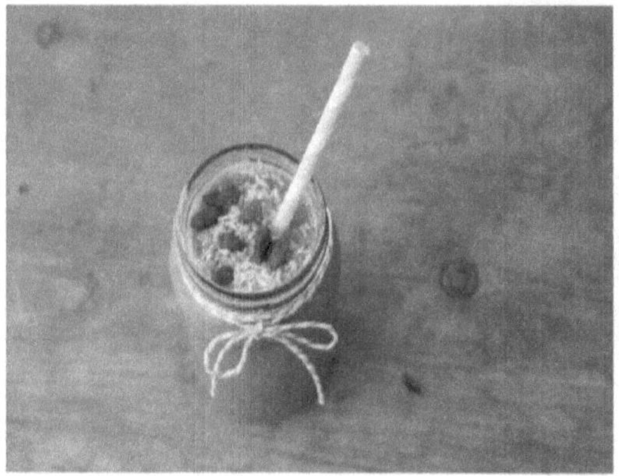

Beet Kale Smoothie

- 1 large beet
- 1 apple
- 1 blood orange
- ½ cup frozen blackberries
- 1 cup kale
- ½ cup crushed ice
- ½ cup water
- 1 tbsp. Hemp Seeds

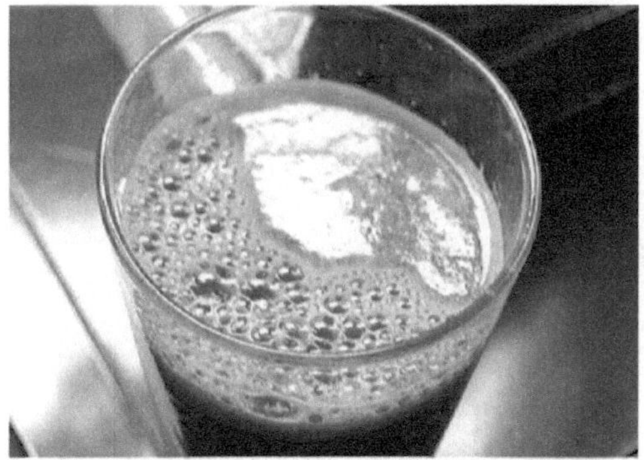

Purple Kale Smoothie

- 1 cup Purple Kale

- 2 apples

- Ginger

- 1 Banana

- 1 cup frozen Blueberries

- 2 tbsp. _Spirulina_

- 1 cup Green tea

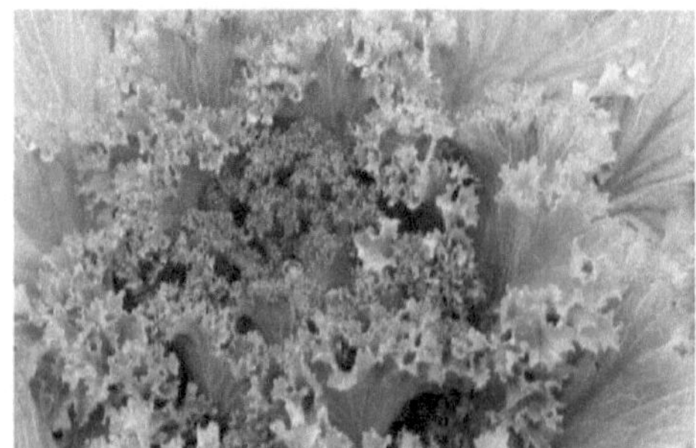

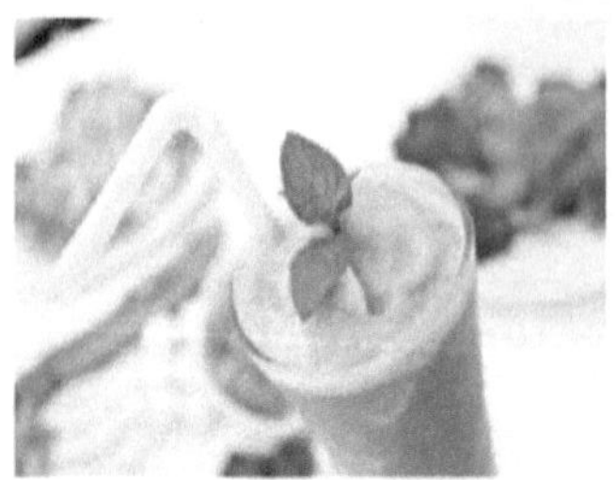

Purple Endive & Fig Smoothie

- 1 cup purple figs

- 1 banana

- 1 cup Purple Belgian Endive

- 1 cup Raspberry leaf tea

- 1 tbsp Chia Seeds

- Top with chopped figs, 1 tbsp. Slivered Almonds and Blueberries

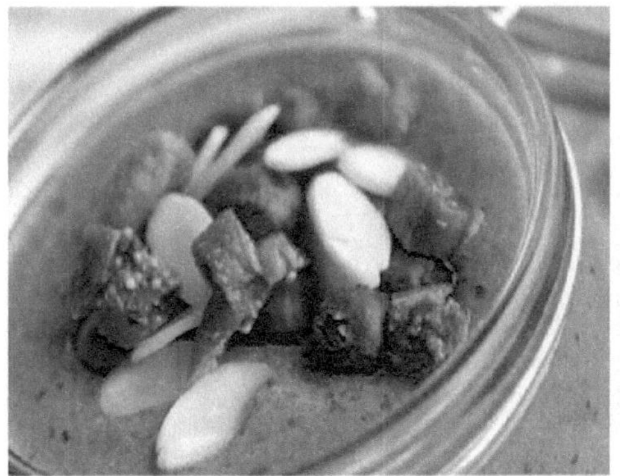

Purple Queen Smoothie

- 2 purple carrots

- 2 tbsp. Almond Butter

- 1 cup Red Dragon fruit (Pitaya)

- 1 tbsp. Maca

- 1 blood Orange

- 1 cup crushed ice

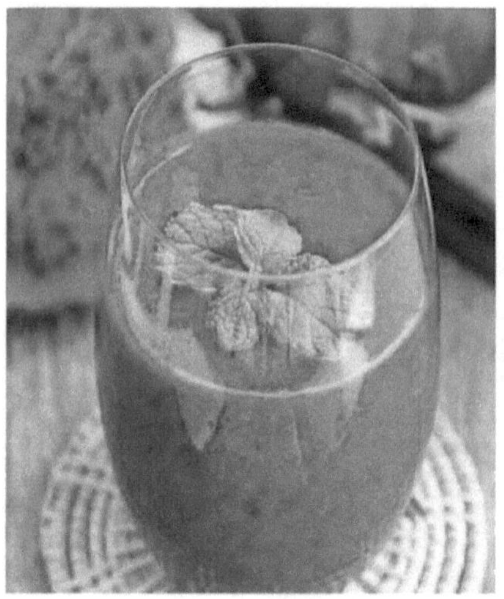

Black Smoothie

- 2 cups spinach
- 1 cup low fat plain yogurt
- 1 banana
- 1/2 cup blueberries, frozen
- 1 cup blackberries, frozen
- 1 tbsp. Cashew nuts
- 1 cup crushed ice

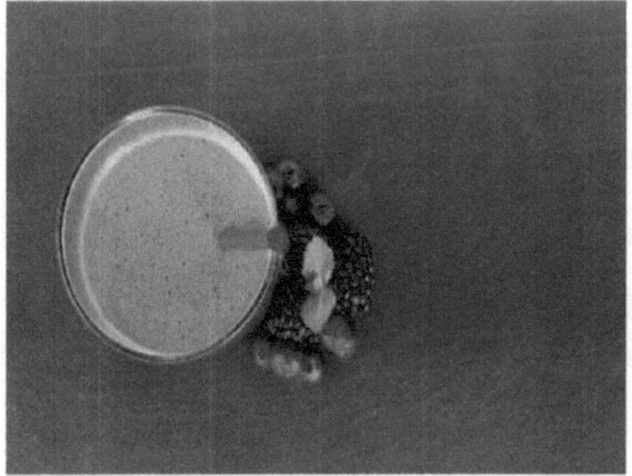

Blueberry Kefir & Spinach Smoothie

• 1 cup blueberries

• 1 cup chopped Cantaloupe

• 1 cup Red Spinach

• 1 cup Green tea

• 1 tbsp. Hemp seeds

• ½ tsp. Cinnamon

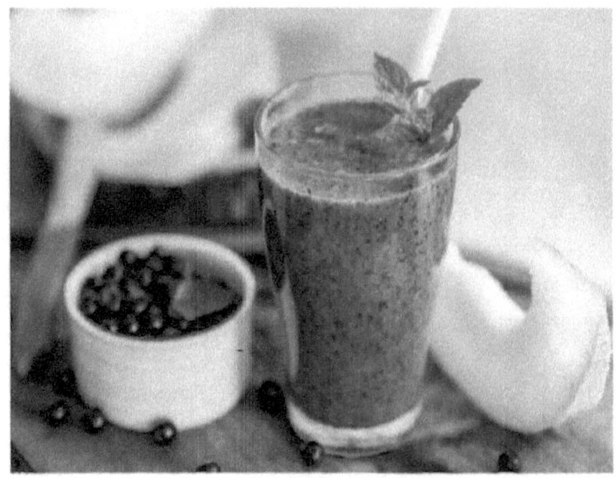

Blackberry Yogurt & Purple Carrots Smoothie

- 1 cup blueberries
- 2 purple carrots
- 1 cup Yogurt
- 1 tbsp. ground _flax_ seeds
- Top with Blackberries

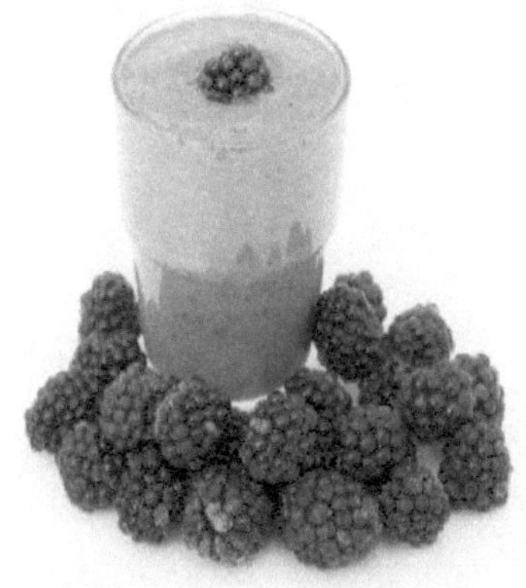

Blackberry, Purple Kale and Mint Smoothie

- 1 cup blackberries

- 1 avocado

- 1 cup Purple Kale

- 1 cup of crushed ice

- 1 tbsp. Chia seeds

- 1 tsp. mint leaves

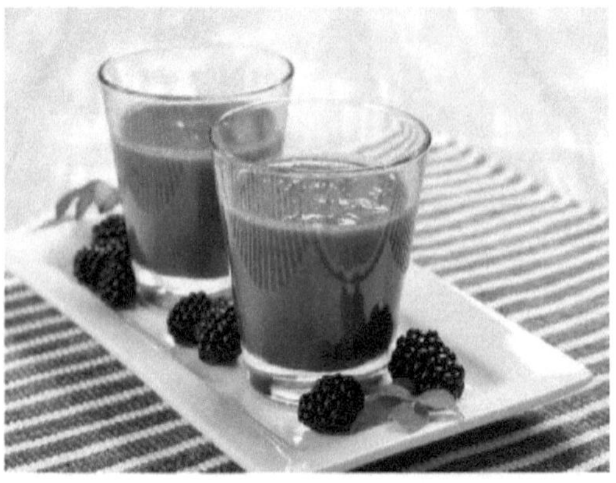

Blackberry Banana Smoothie

- 1 cup blueberries

- 1 banana

- 1 cup of crushed ice

- ½ tsp. Cinnamon

- Top with Blackberries and Banana

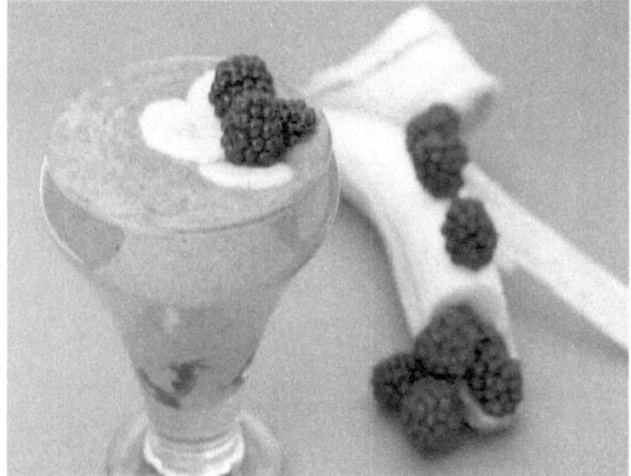

Blueberry & Coconut Smoothie

- 1 cup blueberries

- 1 avocado

- 1 cup Coconut Milk

- 1banana

- ½ tsp. Cinnamon

- Top with Blueberries

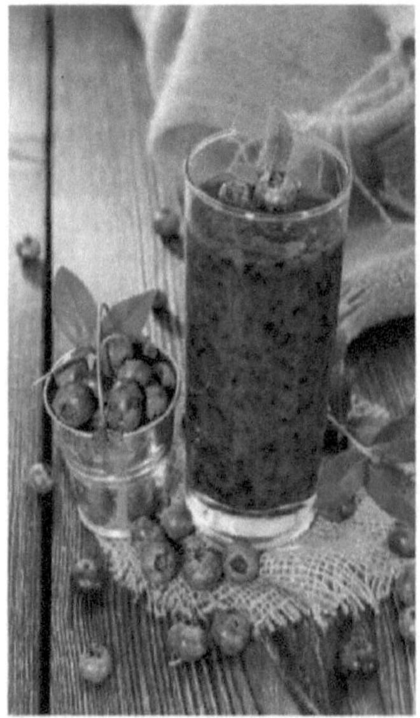

Blueberry, Coconut Flakes & Sesame Seeds Smoothie

- 1 cup blueberries
- 1/2 cup shredded coconut flakes
- 1/2 cup Mulberry
- 1 tbsp. sesame seeds
- 1 cup of crushed ice
- a pinch of nutmeg

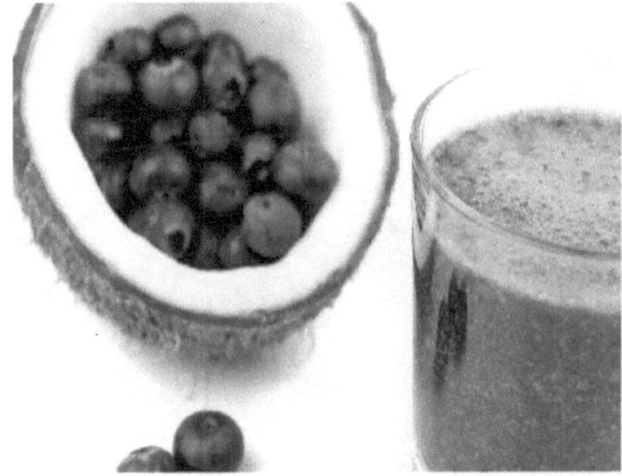

Blueberry & Purple Cauliflower Smoothie

- 1 cup blueberries

- 1 cup Purple Cauliflower

- 1 cup of crushed ice

- 1 banana

- ½ tsp. Cinnamon

- Top with Blueberries

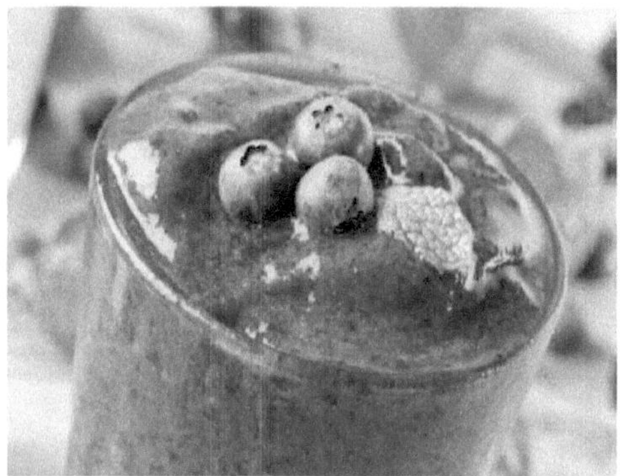

Blueberry & Kefir Smoothie

- 1 cup blueberries

- 1 cup Kefir

- 1/2 cup Raspberries

- ½ tsp. Spirulina

- Top with Blueberries and Mint leaves

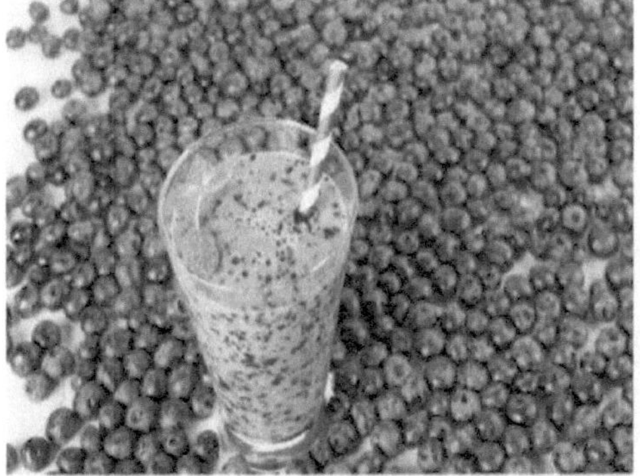

Blueberry & Almond Smoothie

- 1 cup blueberries

- 1 banana

- 1 cup unsweetened Almond Milk

- 1 Tbsp. almond butter

- ½ tsp. Acai

- Top with Blueberries

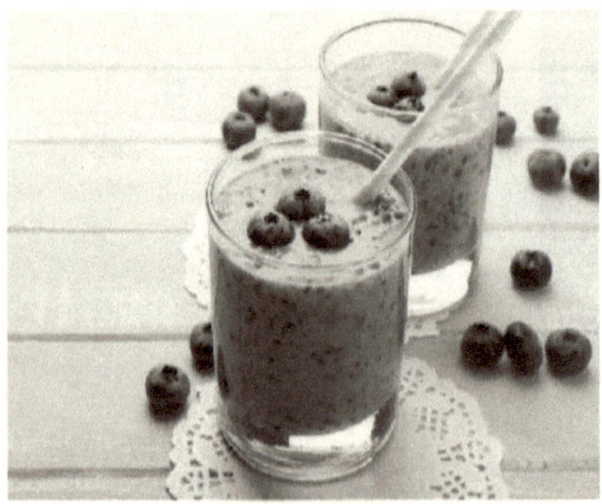

Blueberry & Oatmeal Smoothie

- 1 cup blueberries
- 1 avocado
- 1/2 cup oats
- 2 bananas
- 1 cup of crushed ice
- ½ tsp. Chlorella
- Top with Blueberries and oatmeal flakes

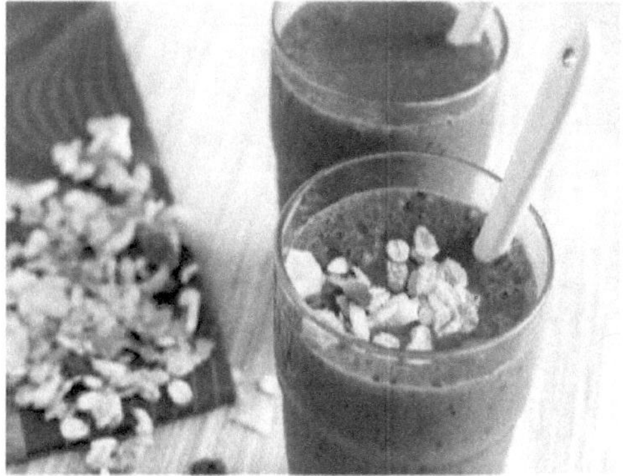

Dragon Fruit & Banana Smoothie

- 1 cup chopped Dragon Fruit

- 1 avocado

- 1 banana

- 1 cup of crushed ice

- 1 tbsp. Chia seeds

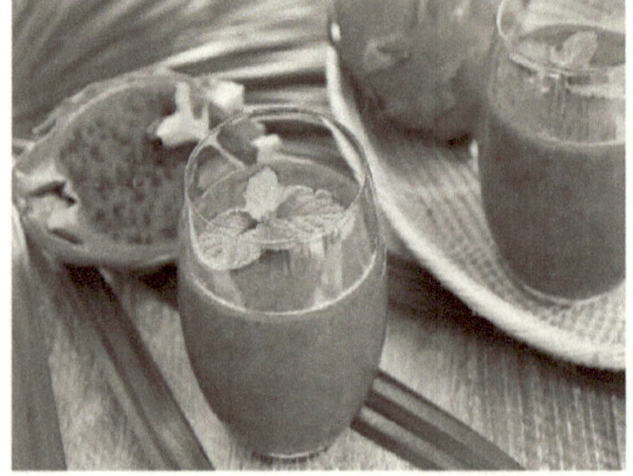

Beet, Broccoli & Apple Smoothie

- 1 cup chopped broccoli
- 1 apple
- 1 cup spinach
- 1 cup of crushed ice
- 1 carrot
- ½ tsp. ginger

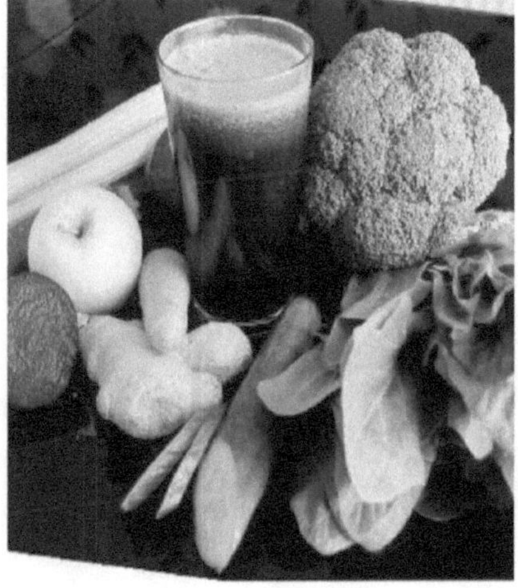

Blueberry & Strawberry Smoothie

- 1 cup blueberries

- 1 cup Strawberries

- 1 banana

- 1 cup of crushed ice

- ½ tsp. <u>Matcha</u>

- Top with Blueberries

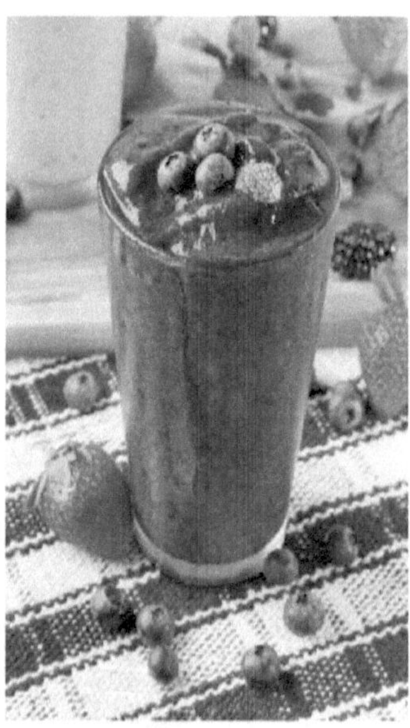

Blueberry, Kefir & Oats Smoothie

- 1 cup blueberries

- 1 cup oats

- 1 cup Kefir

- 1 tbsp. Ground <u>flax</u> seeds

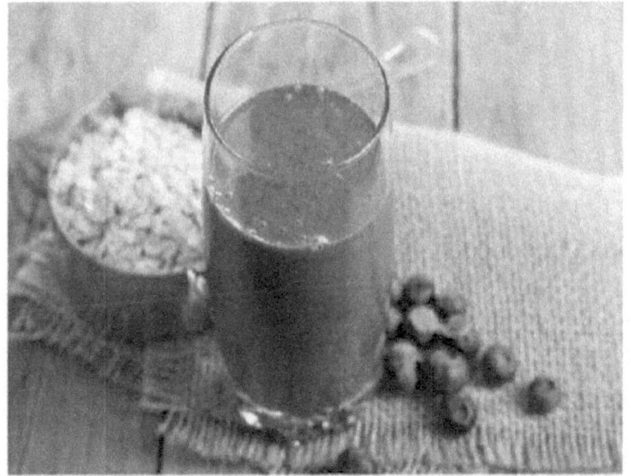

Raspberry, Oats & Blueberry Smoothie

- 1 cup blueberries

- ¼ cup oats

- 1 cup raspberries

- 1 banana

- 1 cup of crushed ice

- 1 tsp. Maqui

- Top with Blueberries and oat flakes

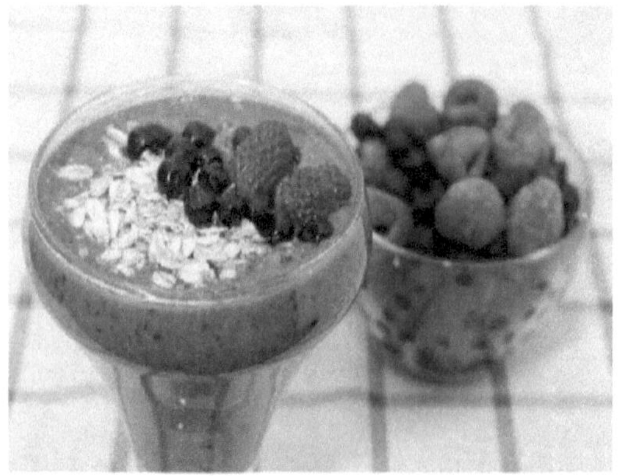

Double Currants Smoothie

- 1 cup Black Currants

- 1 avocado

- 1 cup Red Currants

- 1 cup of crushed ice

- 1 banana

- 1 tbsp. Hemp Hearts

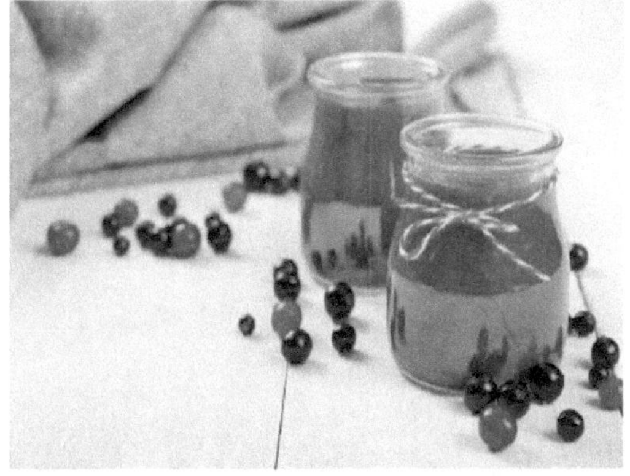

Blueberry & Dandelion Smoothie

- 1 cup blueberries

- 2 bananas

- 1 cup Dandelion

- 1 tbsp. Ground <u>flax</u> seeds

- 1 cup of crushed ice

- ½ tsp. Sesame seeds

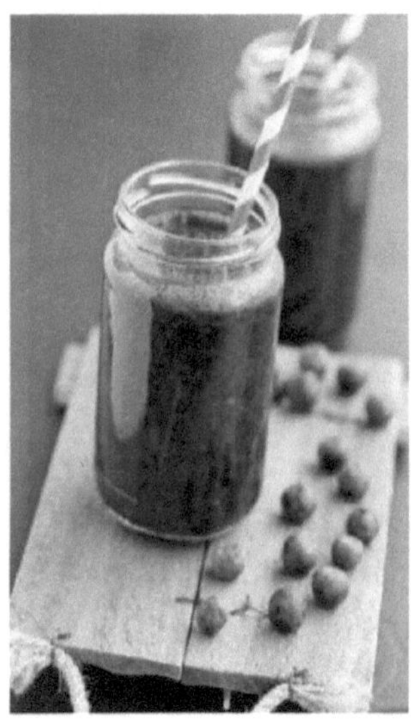

Red Currants, Broccoli & Black Currants Smoothie

- 1 cup Black Currants
- ½ cup broccoli florets
- 1 cup Red Currants
- 1 avocado
- 1 cup of crushed ice
- 1 tsp. Spirulina
- ½ tsp. Cinnamon

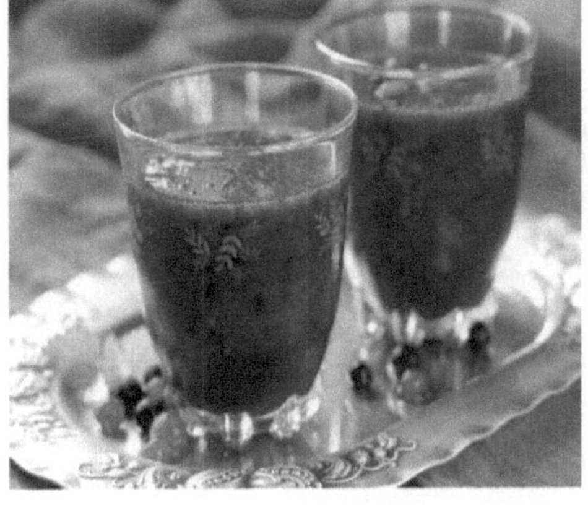

Frozen Berries, Yogurt & Banana Smoothie

- 1 cup mixed frozen Berries

- 2 banana

- 1/2 cup Yogurt

- 1/4 cup Sunflower seeds

- 2 tbsp. Pumpkin seeds

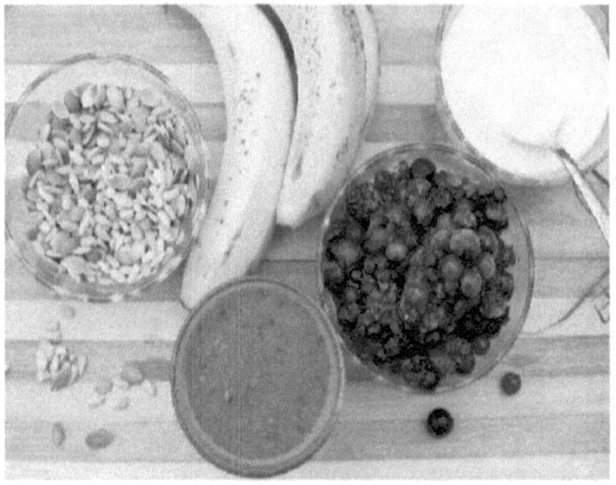

Blueberry, Kefir, Coconut & Oats Smoothie

- 1 cup blueberries

- 1 avocado

- 1/2 cup oats

- 1 cup Kefir

- 1 tbsp. Ground Almond

- ½ tsp. shredded coconut

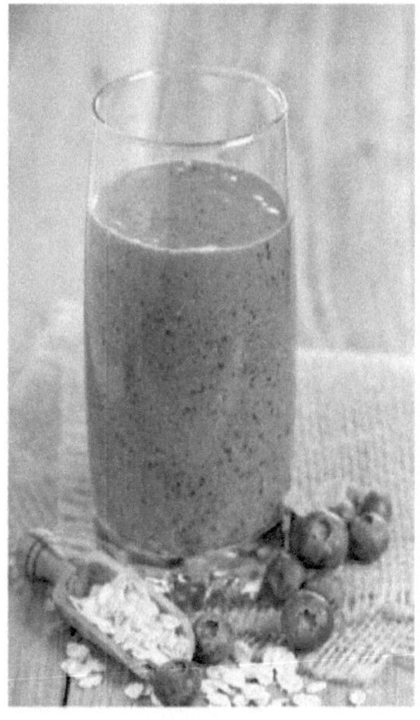

Blueberry Raspberry & Tahini Smoothie

• 1 cup blueberries

• ¼ tahini

• 1 cup Raspberries

• 1 tbsp. Ground <u>flax</u> seeds

• 1 cup of crushed ice

• Top with Blueberries flakes

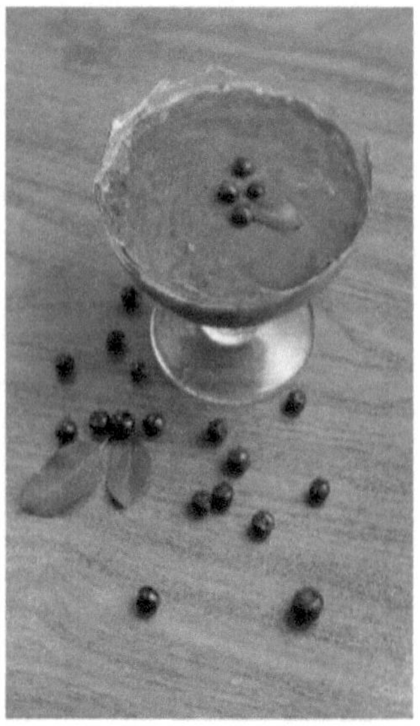

Beet & Kale Smoothie

- 1 cup chopped Kale leaves
- 1 avocado
- 1 cup chopped Beet
- 1 cup of crushed ice
- 2 tsp. raw honey
- 1 banana

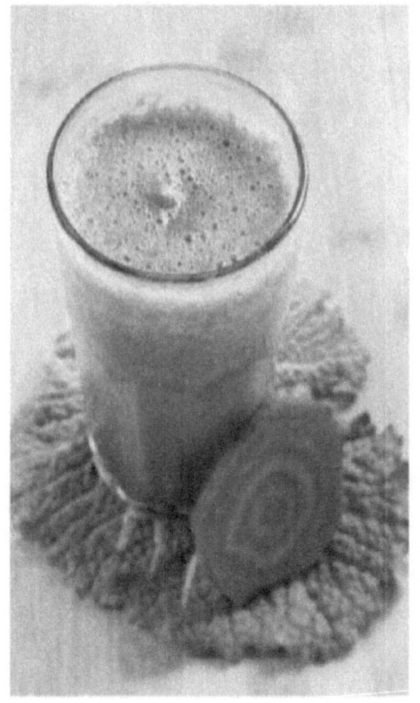

Raspberry, Blueberry & Endive Smoothie

- 1 cup blueberries
- 1 avocado
- 1 cup Raspberries
- 1 cup of crushed ice
- 1/2 cup Endive leaves
- 1 banana
- ½ tsp. Cinnamon
- Top with Blueberries flakes

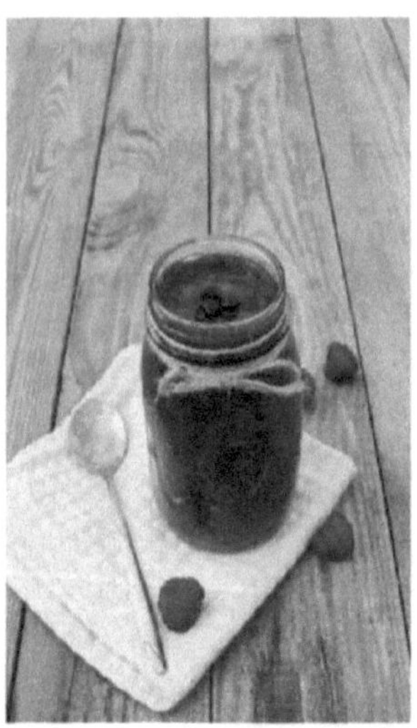

Banana, Chia & Blueberry Smoothie

- 1 cup blueberries

- 2 bananas

- 1 cup of crushed ice

- 1/2 cup Mulberry

- 2 tbsp. Chia seeds

- Top with Blueberries and Coconut flakes

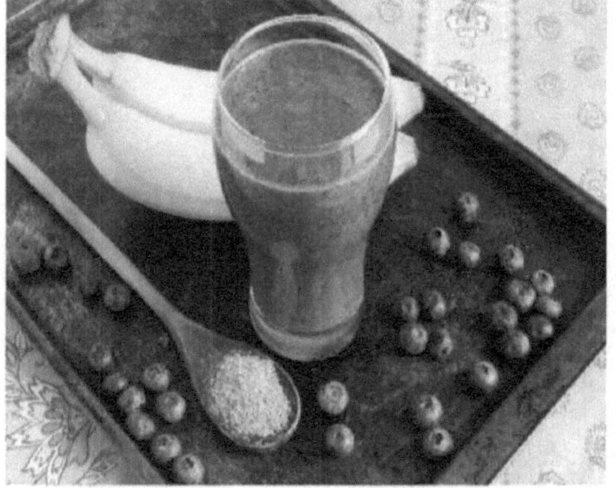

Blackberry, Buttermilk & Mint Smoothie

- 1 cup blackberries

- 1 avocado

- 1 cup Buttermilk

- 1 tbsp. Ground flax seeds

- a pinch of nutmeg

- Top with mint leaves

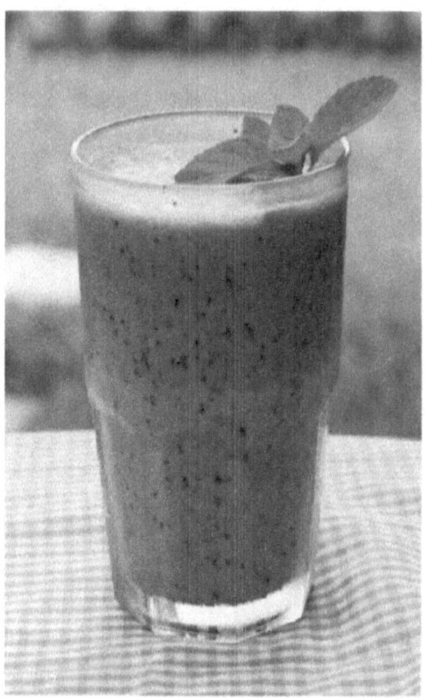

Blueberry Buttermilk & Avocado Smoothie

- 1 cup blueberries

- 1 avocado

- 1 cup Buttermilk

- 1 tbsp. Ground flax seeds

- ½ tsp. Cinnamon

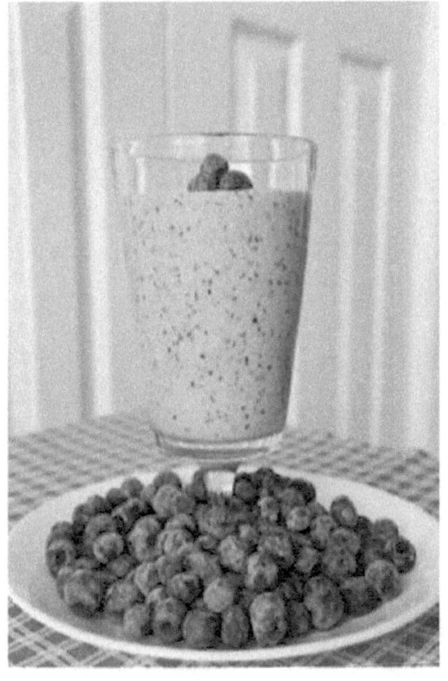

Blueberry Celery Ginger & Apple Smoothie

- 1 cup blueberries
- 1 Apple
- 1 cup Chopped Celery
- 1 cup Yogurt
- 1 Tsp. chopped ginger

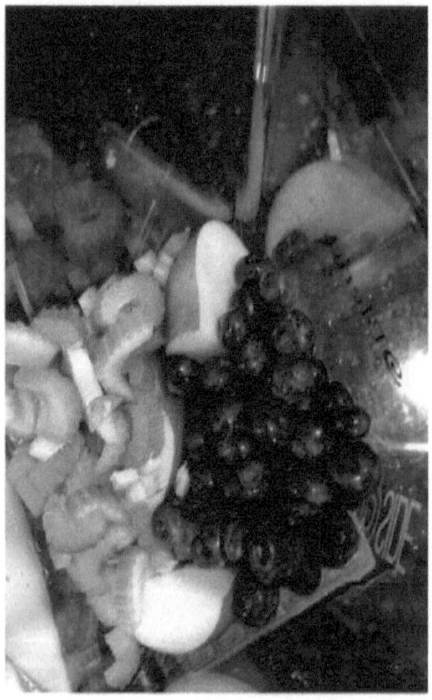

Rainbow Smoothie

3 Colors Rainbow Smoothie

- Blend 1 Large beet with some crushed ice

- Blend 3 carrots with some crashed ice

- Blend 1 cucumber, 1 cup of leaf lettuce, some ice and ½ cup Wheatgrass

- Serve them separate to preserve the distinct color

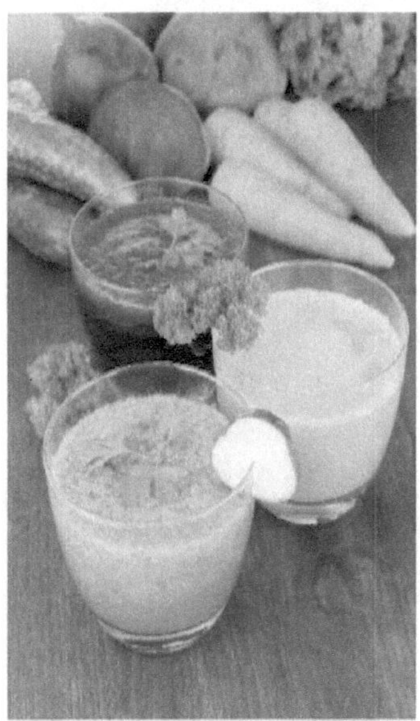

Superfoods Reference Book

Unfortunately, I had to take out the whole Superfoods Reference Book out of all of my books because parts of that book are featured on my blog. I joined Kindle Direct Publishing Select program which allows me to have all my books free for 5 days every 3 months. Unfortunately, KDP Select program also means that all my books have to have unique content that is not available in any other online store or on the Internet (including my blog). I didn't want to remove parts of Superfoods Reference book that is already on my blog because I want that all people have free access to that information. I also wanted to be part of KDP Select program because that is an option to give my book for free to anyone. So, some sections of my Superfoods Reference Book can be found on my blog, under Superfoods menu on my blog. Complete Reference book is available for subscribers to my Superfoods Today Newsletter. Subscribers to my Newsletter will also get information whenever any of my books becomes free on Amazon. I will not offer any product pitches or anything similar to my subscribers, only Superfoods related information, recipes and weight loss and fitness tips. So, subscribe to my newsletter, download Superfoods Cookbook Book Two free eBook which has complete Superfood Reference book included and have the opportunity to get all of my future books for free.

ORAC Value List

ORAC is short for Oxygen Radical Absorbance Capacity. It was developed by the National Institutes of Health in Baltimore.

ORAC units are measurement of the antioxidant capacity of foods. The higher the ORAC value, the more antioxidants the food has.

Foods high in antioxidants lower the risks of cancer and disease.

You'll notice that spices have the most antioxidants. But the ORAC value is measured in dry spices and that is why the values are so high. Common foods such as berries, beans and apples have much fewer antioxidants per gram, because they are full of water. Plus, you can't eat 6 oz. of cloves in one meal, but you can eat 6 oz. of apples. You will notice that e.g. white raisins have higher ORAC value than grape seeds although they are pretty much the same food, but that is because raisins have less water. Every food on this list above value 2 is great. It's better not to pay too much attention to exact ORAC number, just keep eating them all and try to squeeze as much top rated foods as you can. ORAC values in the table are divided per 1000, e.g. Cloves have ORAC rating over 314000, but I slashed 1000 off of each value to keep it easier to compare. Chia seeds are not on this list, but they have value around 6.

1	Cloves, ground	314
2	Sumac bran	312
3	Cinnamon, ground	268
4	Sorghum, bran, raw	240
5	Oregano, dried	200
6	Turmeric, ground	159
7	Acai berry, freeze-dried	103
8	Sorghum, bran, black	101
9	Sumac, grain, raw	87
10	Cocoa powder, unsweetened	81
11	Cumin seed	77
12	Maqui berry, powder	75
13	Parsley, dried	74
14	Sorghum, bran, red	71
15	Basil, dried	68
16	Baking chocolate, unsweetened	50
17	Curry powder	49
18	Sorghum, grain, hi-tannin	45
19	Chocolate, dutched powder	40
20	Maqui berry, juice	40

21	Sage	32
22	Mustard seed, yellow	29
23	Ginger, ground	29
24	Pepper, black	28
25	Thyme, fresh	27
26	Marjoram, fresh	27
27	Goji berries	25
28	Rice bran, crude	24
29	Chili powder	24
30	Sorghum, grain, black	22
31	Chocolate, dark	21
32	Flax hull lignans	20
33	Chocolate, semisweet	18
34	Pecans	18
35	Paprika	18
36	Chokeberry, raw	16
37	Tarragon, fresh	16
38	Ginger root, raw	15
39	Elderberries, raw	15
40	Sorghum, grain, red	14
41	Peppermint, fresh	14
42	Oregano, fresh	14
43	Walnuts	14
44	Hazelnuts	10
45	Cranberries, raw	10
46	Pears, dried	9
47	Savory, fresh	9
48	Artichokes	9
49	Kidney beans, red	8
50	Pink beans	8
51	Black beans	8
52	Pistachio nuts	8
53	Currants	8
54	Pinto beans	8
55	Plums	8
56	Chocolate, milk chocolate	8
57	Lentils	7
58	Agave, dried	7
59	Apples, dried	7
60	Garlic powder	7

61	Blueberries	7
62	Prunes	7
63	Sorghum, bran, white	6
64	Lemon balm, leaves	6
65	Soybeans	6
66	Onion powder	6
67	Blackberries	5
68	Garlic, raw	5
69	Cilantro leaves	5
70	Wine, Cabernet Sauvignon	5
71	Raspberries	5
72	Basil, fresh	5
73	Almonds	4
74	Dill weed	4
75	Cowpeas	4
76	Apples, red delicious	4
77	Peaches, dried	4
78	Raisins, white	4
79	Apples, granny smith	4
80	Dates	4

81	Wine, red	4
82	Strawberries	4
83	Peanut butter, smooth	3
84	Currants, red	3
85	Figs	3
86	Cherries	3
87	Gooseberries	3
88	Apricots, dried	3
89	Peanuts, all types	3
90	Cabbage, red	3
91	Broccoli	3
92	Apples	3
93	Raisins	3
94	Pears	3
95	Agave	3
96	Blueberry juice	3
97	Cardamom	2,7
98	Guava	2,5
99	Lettuce, red leaf	2,38
100	Concord grape juice	2,37

101	Cereals, ready-to-eat, corn flakes	2,36
102	Juice, Pomegranate, 100%	2,34
103	Cereals, oats, instant, fortified, plain, dry	2,31
104	Cereals ready-to-eat, granola, low-fat, with raisins	2,29
105	Cabbage, red, raw	2,25
106	Apples, Golden Delicious, raw, without skin	2,21
107	Sorghum, grain, white	2,20
108	Radish seeds, sprouted, raw	2,18
109	Cereals ready-to-eat, oat bran	2,18
110	Cereals ready-to-eat, toasted oatmeal	2,18
111	Cereals, oats, quick, uncooked	2,17
112	Asparagus, raw	2,15
113	Cereals ready-to-eat, oatmeal, toasted squares	2,14
114	Sweet potato, cooked, baked in skin, without salt	2,12
115	Bread, butternut whole grain	2,10
116	Chives, raw	2,09
117	Cabbage, savoy, cooked, boiled, drained, without salt	2,05
118	Prune juice, canned	2,04
119	Guava, red-fleshed	1,99
120	Applesauce, canned, unsweetened, without added ascorbic acid	1,97
121	Bread, pumpernickel	1,96
122	Nuts, cashew nuts, raw	1,95
123	Beet greens, raw	1,95
124	Avocados, Hass, raw	1,93
125	Pears, green cultivars, with peel, raw	1,91
126	Rocket, raw	1,90
127	Oranges, raw, navels	1,82
128	Peaches, raw	1,81
129	Juice, red grape	1,79
130	Cabbage, black, cooked	1,77
131	Beets, raw	1,77
132	Pears, red anjou, raw	1,75
133	Snacks, popcorn, air-popped	1,74
134	Radishes, raw	1,74
135	Cereals, oats, old fashioned, uncooked	1,71
136	Tortilla chips, reduced fat, Olestra - TEMPORARY	1,70
137	Nuts, macadamia nuts, dry roasted, without salt added	1,70
138	Spinach, frozen, chopped or leaf, unprepared	1,69
139	Potatoes, Russet, flesh and skin, baked	1,68
140	Asparagus, cooked, boiled, drained	1,64

#	Item	Value
141	Tangerines, (mandarin oranges), raw	1,62
142	Broccoli raab, cooked	1,55
143	Grapefruit, raw, pink and red, all areas	1,55
144	Onions, red, raw	1,52
145	Beans, navy, mature seeds, raw	1,52
146	Cereals ready-to-eat, QUAKER, QUAKER OAT LIFE, plain	1,52
147	Spinach, raw	1,52
148	Alfalfa seeds, sprouted, raw	1,51
149	Juice, Cranberry/Concord grape	1,48
150	Lettuce, green leaf, raw	1,45
151	Lettuce, butterhead (includes boston and bibb types), raw	1,42
152	Bread, mixed-grain (includes whole-grain, 7-grain)	1,42
153	Nuts, brazilnuts, dried, unblanched	1,42
154	Broccoli, raw	1,36
155	Potatoes, red, flesh and skin, baked	1,33
156	Potatoes, russet, flesh and skin, raw	1,32
157	Bread, Oatnut	1,32
158	Cereals ready-to-eat, wheat, shredded, plain, sugar and salt free	1,30
159	Parsley, raw	1,30
160	Milk, chocolate, fluid, commercial, reduced fat	1,26
161	Grapes, red, raw	1,26
162	Tea, green, brewed	1,25
163	Agave, raw (Southwest)	1,25
164	Grapefruit juice, white, raw	1,24
165	Lemon juice, raw	1,23
166	Onions, yellow, sauteed	1,22
167	Kiwi, gold, raw	1,21
168	Olive oil, extra-virgin	1,15
169	Potatoes, white, flesh and skin, baked	1,14
170	Tea, brewed, prepared with tap water	1,13
171	Grapes, white or green, raw	1,12
172	Apricots, raw	1,12
173	Potatoes, red, flesh and skin, raw	1,10
174	Potatoes, white, flesh and skin, raw	1,06
175	Onions, raw	1,03
176	Alcoholic beverage, wine, table, rose	1,01
177	Mangos, raw	1,00
178	Juice, strawberry	1,00
179	Sauce, ready-to-serve, salsa	1,00
180	Peppers, sweet, orange, raw	0,98

181	Peppers, sweet, yellow, raw	0,97
182	Lettuce, cos or romaine, raw	0,96
183	Soybeans, mature seeds, sprouted, raw	0,96
184	Eggplant, raw	0,93
185	Peppers, sweet, green, raw	0,92
186	Beans, pinto, mature seeds, cooked, boiled, without salt	0,90
187	Sweet potato, raw, unprepared	0,90
188	Pineapple, raw, extra sweet variety	0,88
189	Kiwi fruit, (chinese gooseberries), fresh, raw	0,88
190	Bananas, raw	0,88
191	Juice, cranberrry, 100% - cranberry blend, red	0,87
192	Onions, white, raw	0,86
193	Cabbage, cooked, boiled, drained, without salt	0,86
194	Chickpeas (garbanzo beans, bengal gram), mature seeds, raw	0,85
195	Peppers, sweet, red, sauteed	0,85
196	Raisins, white, fresh (purchased in Italy)	0,83
197	Cauliflower, raw	0,83
198	Lime juice, raw	0,82
199	Grape juice, white	0,79
200	Peppers, sweet, red, raw	0,79

201	Olive oil, extra-virgin, w/parsley, home prepared	0,77
202	Sweet potato, cooked, boiled, without skin	0,77
203	Beans, snap, green, raw	0,76
204	Nectarines, raw	0,75
205	Peas, yellow, mature seeds, raw	0,74
206	Chilchen (Red Berry Beverage) (Navajo)	0,74
207	Corn, sweet, yellow, raw	0,73
208	Orange juice, raw	0,73
209	Pear juice, all varieties	0,70
210	Peppers, sweet, yellow, grilled	0,69
211	Tomato products, canned, sauce	0,69
212	Mush, blue corn with ash (Navajo)	0,68
213	Olive oil, extra-virgin, w/basil, home prepared	0,68
214	Carrots, raw	0,67
215	Cauliflower, cooked, boiled, drained, without salt	0,62
216	Nuts, pine nuts, dried	0,62
217	Peppers, sweet, green, sauteed	0,62
218	Onions, sweet, raw	0,61
219	Peas, green, frozen, unprepared	0,60
220	Catsup	0,58
221	Pineapple juice, canned, unsweetened, without added ascorbic acid	0,57

222	Vinegar, Apple	0,56
223	Pineapple, raw, traditional varieties	0,56
224	Olive oil, extra-virgin, w/garlic, home prepared	0,56
225	Vegetable juice cocktail, canned	0,55
226	Tomatoes, plum, raw	0,55
227	Peas, split, mature seeds, raw	0,52
228	Corn, sweet, yellow, frozen, kernels cut off cob, unprepared	0,52
229	Cabbage, raw	0,51
230	Celery, raw	0,50
231	Broccoli, frozen, spears, unprepared	0,50
232	Leeks, (bulb and lower leaf-portion), raw	0,49
233	Tomato juice, canned, with salt added	0,49
234	Cocoa mix, powder	0,49
235	Pumpkin, raw	0,48
236	Spices, poppy seed	0,48
237	Lettuce, iceberg (includes crisphead types), raw	0,44
238	Carrots, baby, raw	0,44
239	Peaches, canned, heavy syrup, drained	0,44
240	Babyfood, juice, pear	0,41
241	Corn, sweet, yellow, canned, brine pack, regular pack, solids and liquids	0,41
242	Vinegar, Red wine	0,41
243	Apple juice, canned or bottled, unsweetened, without added ascorbic acid	0,41
244	Tomatoes, red, ripe, cooked	0,41
245	Squash, winter, butternut, raw	0,40
246	Alcoholic beverage, wine, table, white	0,39
247	Pineapple, raw, all varieties	0,39
248	Tomatoes, red, ripe, raw, year round average	0,37
249	Carrots, cooked, boiled, drained, without salt	0,32
250	Melons, cantaloupe, raw	0,32
251	Fennel, bulb, raw	0,31
252	Beans, snap, green variety, canned, regular pack, solids and liquids	0,29
253	Vinegar, Apple and Honey	0,27
254	Eggplant, cooked, boiled, drained, without salt	0,25
255	Beans, lima, immature seeds, canned, regular pack, solids and liquids	0,24
256	Melons, honeydew, raw	0,24
257	Juice, cranberry, white	0,23
258	Vinegar, Honey	0,23
259	Olive oil, extra-virgin, w/garlic and red hot peppers, home prepared	0,22
260	Cucumber, with peel, raw	0,21
261	Squash, summer, zucchini, includes skin, raw	0,18
262	Watermelon, raw	0,14
263	Cucumber, peeled, raw	0,13
264	Oil, peanut, salad or cooking	0,11
265	Limes, raw	0,08